AF580521

CANCER ETIOLOGY, DIAGNOSIS AND TREATMENTS

PROGNOSTIC AND PREDICTIVE RESPONSE THERAPY FACTORS IN CANCER DISEASE

(COLORECTAL, BREAST, LIVER, LUNG, GASTRIC, RENAL AND PROSTATE CANCERS)

CANCER ETIOLOGY, DIAGNOSIS AND TREATMENTS

Additional books in this series can be found on Nova's website under the Series tab.

Additional e-books in this series can be found on Nova's website under the e-book tab.

CANCER ETIOLOGY, DIAGNOSIS AND TREATMENTS

PROGNOSTIC AND PREDICTIVE RESPONSE THERAPY FACTORS IN CANCER DISEASE

(COLORECTAL, BREAST, LIVER, LUNG, GASTRIC, RENAL AND PROSTATE CANCERS)

VINCENZO CANZONIERI
AND
MASSIMILIANO BERRETTA
EDITORS

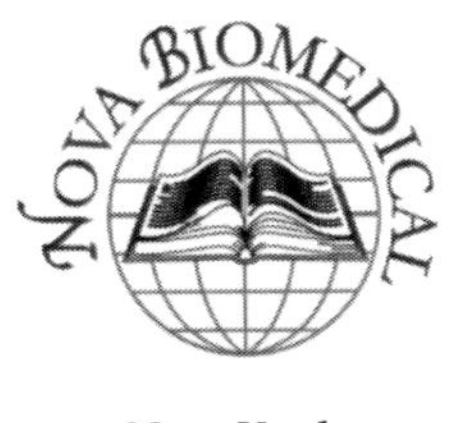

New York

Library of Congress Cataloging-in-Publication Data

ISBN: 978-1-63463-545-5

Library of Congress Control Number: 2014955552

Published by Nova Science Publishers, Inc. † New York

Contents

Preface

The Oncologic science is living a profound change, about diagnostic, prognostic and treatment aspects of cancer disease due to continuous discoveries. Thanks to these new aspects, cancer patients live more and better.

In the recent years we use, in our clinical practice, more informations regarding biological aspects of cancer disease and clinical informations that we can resume as prognostic factors and predictive factors to response oncological medical treatment.

Prognostic tools are important to better understand if cancer patients will have some benefit from antiblastic treatments and to stratify the risk of relapse/progression of cancer disease.

We can divide prognostic tools in Biological and Clinical and often their use in clinical practice is complementary. Recently their use is impacting in clinical practice and due to their role we can personalized antiblastic treatment choosing tailored treatment, according to receptor expression, gene profiles, proliferation index of cancer disease, stage of disease, age, comorbities and PS.

We think that their appropriate use is the right way to have better response rate by antiblastic treatments, to reduce toxicities and final to choose the right drug save economic resources.

Also in the fields of pathology the relevance of prognosis in cancer and the prediction of treatment response represent an invaluable set of information provided by the pathologist by using molecular approaches both in situ and in liquid phase, such as immunohistochemistry, in situ hybridization, mutational status assessment for therapeutic relevant genes.

Of importance are, in this context, the problems of quantitation and standardization of methods, techniques and interpretation of results. The

Pathological Societies are constantly involved in the elaboration of guidelines and definition of cut-offs and we believe that this is one of the fields of medicine that is more exposed to continuous evolution.

The pathological assessment in oncology have to be accurate, prompt and clinical relevant. Today, this is referred not only to aspects of modern and sophisticated diagnostic process and tumor staging, but also to tumor prognostication and definition of the best treatment.

In: Prognostic and Predictive Response ... ISBN: 978-1-63463-545-5
Editors: V. Canzonieri and M. Berretta

Chapter 1

Breast Cancer: Prognostic and Predictive Response Therapy Factors

Tiziana Perin[1*], Simon Spazzapan[2], Valentina Guida[1], Massimiliano Berretta[3], Gustavo Baldassarre[4] and Vincenzo Canzonieri[1]

[1,4]Division of Experimental Oncology, CRO - National Cancer Institute, IRCCS Aviano, Italy

[2,3]Medical Oncology C CRO - National Cancer Institute, IRCCS Aviano, Italy

Abstract

Because of the rapid progression of breast cancer (BC) through the intermediate stage up until invasive and then metastatic carcinoma, the identification of prognostic and predictive factors is vital. One of the causes of breast cancer development is multiple gene mutations that lead to molecular abnormalities. Here we review the clinical, serum, and tissue biomarkers and the use of innovative prognostic factors. Clinical follow-

* Corresponding author: Tiziana Perin, Division of Pathology, National Cancer Istitute. I.R.C.C.S., Via F. Gallini 2 Aviano (PN), 33081 Italy, Phone +39 434659625, tperin@cro.it.

up in BC stands a chance to have appropriate therapies that limit the toxicity and side effects of treatment and to provide physical and psychosocial support.

In the era of genomic sequencing and sub-classification of cancers, novel strategies have been developed to assess the prognosis of breast cancer; however, these new tools have not yet been integrated into the surveillance strategies. Hopefully, in the near future, not only target therapies, but also personalized follow-up visits will be available. Before this becomes a reality, however, new studies are needed.

Introduction

Breast cancer is the most common tumor among the women of developed countries and the developing world. Even though there have been advancements in medical research concerning the treatment of breast cancer and the possibility of early diagnosis thanks to prevention, breast cancer is the second leading cause of female death after pulmonary cancer. Several etiological factors have been implicated in its pathogenesis: age, genetics, family history, pregnancy, obesity, lifestyle, co-morbidities, and endocrine factors (both endogenous and exogenous).

Breast cancer is a heterogeneous disease, and it is divided into subgroups according to histo-morphological characteristics (such as histological subtype and grading), TNM staging information (tumor size, T; lymph node, N; distant metastasis occurrence, M), and gene expression profiling. Genetic studies have identified unique molecular patterns for each subgroup of breast cancer according to the expression of hormone receptors (estrogen and progesterone receptors), human epidermal growth factor receptors (HER), anti-apoptosis markers (p53), cell proliferation indicators (Ki-67), Keratins (CK) expressions, epithelial to mesenchymal transitions (EMT), microRNAs or other non-coding RNAs, and regulating factors. Each molecular pattern seems to be linked to specific prognosis and seems to be the consequence of a specific pathogenesis. Implementation of molecular subgrouping is important for the treatment of breast cancer: different therapeutic approaches are possible on the strength of the receptors and target expression by tumor cells. In breast cancer, hormonal or “target therapy” is possible if estrogen (ER) and/or progesterone receptors (PgR) and HER-2 are respectively expressed. Thanks to hormone therapy (e.g. tamoxifen) and “target therapy” (e.g. trastuzumab, lapatinib), a better response to drug treatments and higher survival, both disease free (DSF) and overall (OS), are obtained in patients with breast carcinoma. The appropriate therapeutic approach for breast cancer patients is possible thanks to the use of validated prognostic and predictive factors. The prognostic factor provides information on clinical outcome independent of treatment, whereas predictive factor is associated with response to a given therapy. The determination of prognostic and predictive markers is a useful tool for clinical management in cancer patients and in the development of new treatment modalities.

Clinical Prognostic Factors

In 2008, the estimated age-adjusted annual incidence of breast cancer in Europe (40 countries) was 88.4/100.000 and the mortality 24.3/100.000[1]. The overall burden of breast cancer in the developing world is growing as a consequence of Westernization, lowering age of menarche, declining fertility, and last but not least, the increase in life expectancy.

Age

There is a steep age gradient with about a quarter of breast cancers occurring before age 50 and <5% before age 35 [2]. Thus, age by itself is a classical risk factor, but it may be also a prognostic factor.

The issue is clinically relevant because, if age is an independent prognostic factor, then young women with breast cancer might benefit from treatments other than those offered to older women with the same tumor profile. In this context, it would be interesting to understand if the dismal outcome seen in breast cancer patients under the age of 40 is due to premenopausal status or to a major frequency of less favorable pathological features in younger women.

However, age per se is a strong risk factor in premenopausal breast cancer patients [3] after also adjusting for other prognostic factors [4]. The risk for breast cancer recurrence for women diagnosed below the age of 40 has been estimated to be 1.53-fold higher than the risk for those diagnosed at 40 years or older (95% CI 1.37-1.74) [4].

Pregnancy

Ten percent of breast cancer cases diagnosed in patients below the age of 40 in Western nations are pregnancy–associated breast cancer, commonly defined as breast cancer diagnosed during the course of pregnancy or the one-year period following delivery [5]. The relative rarity of this disease precludes the conductions of large-powered controlled studies, so the prognosis is not well-defined.

Some studies have found an independent effect of pregnancy on outcome [6, 7, 8], and others have found that pregnancy-associated breast cancer is more commonly diagnosed at an advanced stage, suggesting a poorer prognosis due to a diagnostic delay [9, 10].

Pregnancy–associated breast cancer was found to be a negative prognostic factor in a comprehensive analysis of all published studies. A clearer trend of poorer outcomes was seen in those diagnosed postpartum (pHR: 1.84; 95% CI (1.28-2.65) than in those diagnosed during pregnancy [11].

Obesity

In Europe, the prevalence of obesity (body mass index (BMI) ≥ 30 kg/m2) in men ranged from 4.0% to 8.3% and in women from 6.2% to 36.5% [12].

Obesity was a negative prognostic factor in a recent meta-analysis, including 43 studies that enrolled women diagnosed with breast cancer between 1963 and 2005 [13].

Obesity (BMI>30 kg/m^2) was associated with inferior outcomes, especially in postmenopausal hormone receptor positive operable breast cancer in three adjuvant trials coordinated by ECOG, including E1199, E5188, and E3189, and conducted before trastuzumab therapy. Disease-free survival (HR 1.31; 95% CI, 1.12-1.53; P 0.009) and overall survival (HR 1.46; 95% CI 1.21-1.77; P 0.0001) were statistically significantly inferior in obese versus non-obese patients in ER+ PR+ HER2-. This relation was not observed, however, in triple negative or HER2+ disease [14].

The Comorbidity and Polypharmacy

Late mortality also depends in large part on the impact of comorbidities, especially in older patients. In the USA, as in most Western countries, hypertension, diabetes, mental disorders, and obesity are common in aging patients and have prevalence rates of about 46%, 20%, 31%, and 6%, respectively, in breast cancer patients [15, 16].

Several studies have demonstrated an association between cancer, comorbidities, and outcomes.

In a longitudinal observational study carried out in the Detroit metropolitan area among women aged 40-84 years, patients with three or more comorbidities had a 20-fold higher rate of mortality from causes other than breast cancer and a 4-fold higher rate of all-cause mortality when compared to patients without comorbidity [17].

The hazard ratio for dying for patients with high-grade comorbidities was almost three times higher in a study conducted in Holland by Houterman [18].

There has been a steadily increasing trend of polypharmacy in the geriatric population during the last 20 years. More than 40% of persons aged 65 and older use five or more different medications per week, and 12% use 10 or more different medications [19].

Polypharmacy in older people is associated with impaired physical function and being pre-frail and frail compared to being robust [20], and it is significantly associated with chemotherapy-related toxicity in metastatic breast cancer patients [21].

Inflammatory Breast Cancer

Inflammatory breast cancer (IBC) is rare (5% of breast cancers) but represents the most aggressive form of the disease. Major diagnostic criteria are rapid onset (<6 months) of breast erythema, edema, and/or peau d'orange skin, and/or warm breast, with or without an underlying palpable mass [22]. The characteristic clinical features of inflammatory breast cancer are due to blockage of dermal lymphatics by tumor emboli and not to "inflammation."

Inflammatory breast cancer is usually hormone receptor negative and often HER2 positive. Studies on gene expression profiling of IBC have demonstrated that all the subtypes of inflammatory breast cancers exist, but basal and HER2 overexpressed are more frequent (Network NCC NCCN Clinical Practice Guidelines Invasive Breast Cancer Version I.2014).

The majority of women with IBC have loco-regional disease at diagnosis, and 30% have stage IV de novo disease [23]. The standard treatment option for all patients diagnosed with IBC is primary systemic chemotherapy plus anti-HER2 therapy according to HER2 status followed by a modified radical mastectomy, post-surgery radiation therapy, and hormone treatment if hormone receptor positive [22]. Despite multidisciplinary treatment, 5-year overall survival remains in the range of 40% [24].

Prognostic Serum Markers

The ideal serum tumor marker should be able to (i) detect disease early; (ii) predict response or resistance to specific therapies; and (iii) monitor the patient after primary therapy [25].

CEA, a member of the immunoglobulin superfamily, and CA15.3—the soluble form of MUC-1protein, that is, a large type I transmembrane glycoprotein—are the most frequently used serum tumor markers in breast cancer [26]. They are economic and non-invasive tests; however, they do not respond to the requests of an ideal tumor marker. Their routine use in an otherwise asymptomatic patient with no specific findings on clinical examination during follow-up is generally not recommended [27].

However, rising CA15.3 and CEA have been demonstrated to be able to identify novel relapses before symptoms develop and before traditional radiologic exams [28], and their use may select patients for more sensible and specific exams, such as PET/ct [29].

CEA and CA15-3 may be useful for monitoring the response to therapy in the metastatic phase, particularly in those patients with only bone lesions that are difficult to measure with traditional exams. However, a change in tumor markers alone should not be used as the only determinant for treatment decisions [30].

Due to these diagnostic gaps, several research groups have tried to research new serum tumor markers. The most promising of them are circulating noncoding molecules of RNA (miRNAs). They are found aberrantly expressed in different human cancers and have shown high levels of sensibility and specificity; however, novel large studies are needed before these markers are used in clinical practice [26].

Prognostic and Predective Tissue Factors and Clinical Factors

Breast cancer amounts to approximately 26% of all annually diagnosed cancers and represents the second leading cause of female death after pulmonary cancer. A decline in the incidence rate was recently reported and is largely due to the reduction in the use of hormone replacement therapy [31, 32, 33]. Over the past two decades, the mortality rate has declined significantly, primarily due to the early use of adjuvant systemic therapy as well as detection of earlier stage tumors due to increased screening programs [34, 35].

The mainstay of treatment for patients with localized disease is surgical excision and staging axillary lymph node evaluation with or without radiation therapy. Some patients receive neoadjuvant chemotherapy or hormonal therapy prior to definitive excision of the tumor, mainly in locally advanced tumors. Other treatment options include adjuvant chemotherapy, hormonal therapy, or monoclonal antibodies therapy with a primary goal of eliminating or delaying the subsequent appearance of clinically occult micrometastases.

Thanks to prognostic and predictive factors, we can stratify patients into two groups: one, those who are expected to derive the most benefit from adjuvant systemic therapy, which includes all patients with lymph node metastases and a subset of node-negative patients; and two, those for which the risks and costs of adjuvant therapy outweigh the expected benefits [36].

A prognostic factor may be defined as a measurable variable that correlates with the natural history of the disease: it discriminates patients at low risk, for whom the adjuvant therapy is not indicated, and patients at higher risk who would most benefit from different forms of treatments. A prognostic factor has significant and independent value, validated by clinical testing. Its determination must be feasible, reproducible, and widely available with quality controls. In contrast, a predictive factor is one that is associated with response to a given therapy or improved outcomes as overall survival.

Under the auspices of the College of American Pathologists (CAP), a multidisciplinary group of clinicians, pathologists, and statisticians considered prognostic and predictive factors in breast cancer [37]:

- The presence or the absence of axillary lymph node involvement: Only 20% to 30% of node-negative patients will develop recurrence within 10 years, compared with about 70% of patients with axillary nodal involvement. Patients with 4 or more involved nodes have a worse prognosis than those with fewer than 4 involved nodes [37].
- *Micrometastases:* Defined as < 2 mm in diameter; macrometastases, >0.2 cm in size, have clearly been shown to have prognostic significance.
- *Tumor size:* The frequency of nodal metastases in patients with tumors smaller than 1.0 cm is 10% to 20%, and node-negative patients

with tumors smaller than 1.0 cm have a 10-year disease-free survival rate of about 90% [37].

- *Sentinel lymphadenectomy*: Axillary dissection is generally considered a staging procedure, but may have therapeutic benefit for some patients.
- *Lymphatic/vascular invasion*: Peritumoral vascular invasion (either blood vessel or lymphatic channel) is predictive of local failure and reduced overall survival [37].
- *Histological grade and type of the tumor*: Many breast cancers have a lobular-type, single file, or targetoid growth pattern, but only those with very low-grade nuclei and low cell density are associated with a better prognosis than ordinary breast cancer or other subtypes of invasive lobular carcinoma; tubular and mucinous carcinoma (90% pure) have a particularly favorable prognosis [37].
- *Mitotic index*: Mitotic index is the number of mitotic figures in a given area of tumor, and high mitotic rates have been correlated with poor clinical outcomes [37].
- *Hormone receptor status* (estrogen and progesterone receptors).
- HER2/neu.
- *p53*: Associated with high histologic grade and clinical aggressiveness, and mutation in p53 gene is associated with poor outcomes.
- Proliferation marker (Ki-67).

The American Society of Clinical Pathologists (ASCO) and College of American Pathologists (CAP) recently published guidelines for hormone receptor testing and HER2/neu testing routinely used in clinical practice.

Estrogen Receptor Alpha and Progesterone Receptor

The estrogen receptor-alpha (ER-α) and progesterone receptor are both prognostic and predictive biomarkers for response to endocrine therapy [38, 39]. ER-α is a nuclear transcription factor activated by the hormone estrogen to regulate the development, growth, and differentiation of normal breast tissue [40, 41]. These pathways remain active to varying degrees in invasive breast cancers, including estrogen-stimulated growth of tumor epithelial cells expressing ER-α, which can be detrimental to patients.

Thanks to the use of biochemical ligand-binding assays (LBAs) on tumor breast tissue, in early 1990s, it was demonstrated that ER-α was a weak prognostic factor but a very predictive factor for response to endocrine therapies, such as tamoxifen [42]. Tamoxifen binds ER-α, inhibits the estrogen-stimulated growth of tumor cells and so: reduces cancer recurrences, prolongs survival in patients with ER-α-positive invasive breast cancer [42-47], reduces subsequent breast cancer incidence in patients with ER-α-positive ductal carcinoma in situ [48] and in patients with a high risk for developing breast cancer [49]

The clinical response to aromatase inhibitors (e.g., anastrozole, letrozole, exemestane), which suppress the production of estrogen, is also dependent on the status of ER-α, and only positive tumors benefit [50-53]. The expression of progesterone receptor (PgR) is regulated by ER-α, so the presence of PgR usually indicates that the ER- α pathway is functionally intact. PgR is activated by hormone progesterone to help regulate several normal cell functions, including proliferation.

Thanks to LBA PgR also was demonstrated to be a weak prognostic factor, but a relatively strong predictive factor for response to endocrine therapies. To measure ER-α and PgR in breast tissues, IHC (immunohistochemistry) is used on FFPET (formalin-fixed paraffin-embedded tissue) samples: this method was approved in the 1990s by the CAP and ASCO for routine clinical testing [44], recommending that specific IHC assays must be rigorously standardized and validated in order to be used. Studies evaluating ER-α by IHC in breast cancer demonstrate that about 75%-80% express ER-α that is nuclear in location. Those evaluating PgR in breast cancer demonstrate that about 60%-70% express PgR in a nuclear location.

Both ER-α and PgR expression vary on a continuum ranging from 0% to nearly 100% positive cells (Figures 1 and 2). More importantly, they show a direct correlation between the likelihood of clinical response to endocrine therapies and levels of ER-α and PgR: any tumor expressing very low levels of ER-α or PgR-positive cells (but ≥1%) shows a significant clinical benefit. Thus, the ASCO/CAP guidelines recommend a cut point of 1% or greater IHC- positive cells to define ER-α or PgR positive: we have a positive case for ER or PgR if ≥1% of tumor cell nuclei are immunoreactive, and we have a negative case for ER or PgR if <1% of tumor cell nuclei are immunoreactive in the presence of positive controls.

PgR expression is reduced in patients with DCIS treated with lumpectomy and radiation followed by endocrine therapy [48]. According to ASCO/CAP guidelines, the samples for ER and PgR testing should be fixed in 10% NBF (neutral buffered formalin) for 6 to 72 hours. PgR expression is not perfectly correlated with ER-α: there are four possible phenotypes of combined expression, each with different rates of response to hormonal therapy.

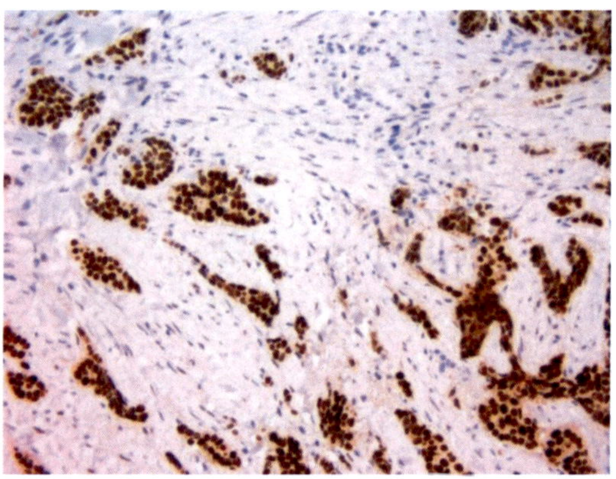

Figure 1. Strong nuclear expression of ERs-alpha in 100% of the tumor cells.

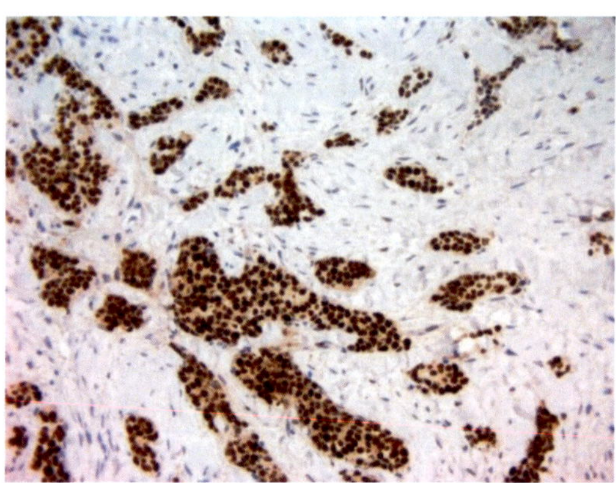

Figure 2. Strong nuclear expression of Progesterone Receptors in 100% of the tumor cells.

In PgR-negative tumors, there is both a nuclear location and an outer cell membrane location of ER-α: these tumors are HER-2 positive, and membrane ER-α promotes tumor cell proliferation in cooperation with overexpressed HER-2 due to non-functional nuclear ER-α [56,57].

HER2/neu (ERBB2)

HER2/neu oncogene is a member of erb-like oncogene family, and it is related to human epidermal growth factor receptor. Upon phosphorylation of MAPK, EGFR signaling regulates the transportation of mitogenic signals across the cell membrane via a signaling cascade. Once intracellular, these signals induce proliferation and inhibit cell death; thus, misregulation of this pathway results in uncontrolled growth and inhibition of apoptosis.

The HER2 gene is overexpressed, and/or protein is amplified in 15%-20% of breast cancer patients [58, 59]. HER2 positive breast cancer has a worse prognosis with a higher rate of recurrence and mortality and is associated with high histological grade and young age. An important aspect of determining HER2 status is also its role as a predictive factor. HER2 positivity is predictive of response to anthracycline- and taxane-based therapy and of relative resistance to all endocrine therapies.

Trastuzumab [60], lapatinib, pertuzumab, and ado-trastuzumab emtansine (T-DM1) [61] have been shown to be effective in the adjuvant setting for women with HER2-positive breast cancer: lapatinib decreases breast cancer cell proliferation in ER-negative tumors and in DCIS and ductal hyperplasia lesions [62]; trastuzumab improves response rates, time to progression, and survival when used alone or associated with chemotherapy; pertuzumab significantly prolonged progression-free survival when used as first-line in the metastatic setting; T-DM1 is a drug with minimal toxicity and significant efficacy in previously treated HER2-overexpressing breast cancer patients.

The humanized HER2 antibody trastuzumab targets the extracellular domain of HER2, while lapatinib inhibits the kinase activity of HER2 and EGFR. Pertuzumab works to block the heterodimerization of HER2 with other HER family members, inhibiting some proteins kinases and promoting antibody-dependent cytotoxicity [62]. T-DM1 is linked to trastuzumab and inhibits microtubule assembly and, thereby, mitosis. Amplification and/or overexpression of the HER2/neu gene are routinely evaluated, using IHC and/or in-situ hybridization (ISH), in all cases of breast carcinoma (early stage or metastatic disease).

The American Society of Clinical Oncology (ASCO) and the College of American Pathologists (CAP) recently published a clinical practice guideline on improving the accuracy of HER2 testing for breast cancer patients [63]: the importance of this guideline is that it ensures that the right patient receives the right treatment. According to the ASCO/CAP guideline, the samples for HER2 testing should be fixed in 10% NBF for 6 to 72 hours. Testing criteria define

HER2-positive status when (on observing within an area of tumor that amounts to >10% of contiguous and homogeneous tumor cells) there is evidence of protein overexpression (IHC) or gene amplification (HER2 copy number or HER2/CEP17 ratio by ISH based on counting at least 20 cells within the area). Further experience with established HER2 assays also led to the identification of unusual HER2 genotypic abnormalities, such as aneusomy of chromosome 17 (polysomy and monosomy), co-localization of HER2 and CEP17 signals that affect HER2/CEP17 ratio in dualsignal in situ hybridization (ISH) assays, and genomic heterogeneity. If results are equivocal (revised criteria), reflex testing should be performed using an alternative assay (IHC or ISH).

HER2 testing by validated IHC assays (Figs. 3, 4, 5) can be:

- IHC 3+ positive: Circumferential membrane staining that is complete, intense, and within > 10% of tumor cells.
- IHC 2+ equivocal: Circumferential membrane staining that is incomplete and/or weak/moderate and within > 10% of tumor cells or complete and circumferential membrane staining that is intense and within ≤ 10% of tumor cells.
- IHC 1+ negative: Incomplete membrane staining that is faint/barely perceptible and within > 10% of tumor cells.
- IHC 0 negative: No staining is observed or membrane staining that is incomplete and is faint/barely perceptible and within ≤ 10% of tumor cells

HER2 testing by validated single-probe ISH assays can be:

- ISH positive: Average HER2 copy number ≥ 6.0 signals/cell.
- ISH equivocal: Average HER2 copy number ≥ 4.0 and < 6.0 signals/cell.
- ISH negative: Average HER2 copy number < 4.0 signals/cell.

HER2 testing (invasive component) by validated dual-probe ISH assay can be:

- ISH positive if:
  - HER2/CEP17 ratio ≥ 2.0: Average HER2 copy number ≥ 4.0 signals/cell.

  - HER2/CEP17 ratio $\geq$ 2.0: Average HER2 copy number < 4.0 signals/cell.
  - HER2/CEP17 ratio < 2.0: Average HER2 copy number $\geq$ 6.0 signals/cell.
- ISH equivocal if:
  - HER2/CEP17 ratio < 2.0: Average HER2 copy number $\geq$ 4.0 and <6.0 signals/cell.
- ISH negative if:
  - HER2/CEP17 ratio < 2.0: Average HER2 copy number < 4.0 signals/cell (Figure 5).

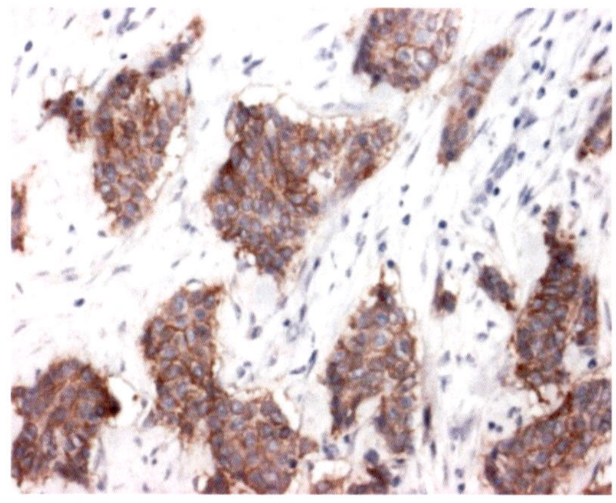

Figure 3. HER-2 positivity, score 2+.

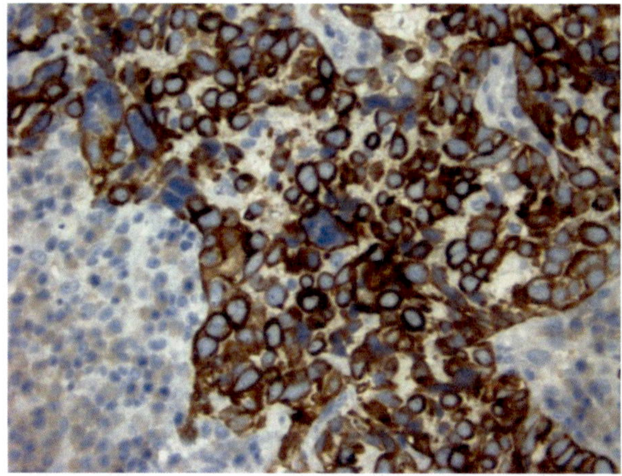

Figure 4. HER-2 positivity, score 3+.

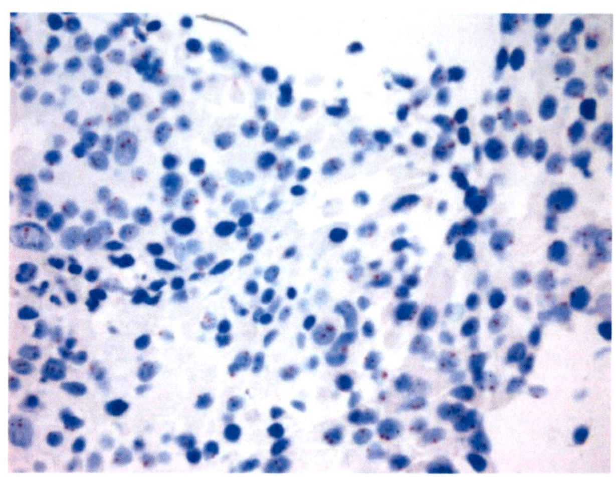

Figure 5. Dual color SISH HER2/CEP17: non amplified.

KI-67

Ki-67 is a nuclear protein associated with cellular proliferation, and it was shown that it is expressed in all phases of the cell cycle other than the G0 phase [64]. Ki-67 antigen expression is often quantified in terms of percentage of positively stained cells among the total number of malignant cells scored. This is usually a semi-quantitative estimate determined by pathologists, who count as many as 500-1000 nuclei to determine this proportion.

Another potential source of variability in this measurement is the field of view (FOV) selected by the pathologist for determining Ki-67 [70]. The most widely used method to detect Ki-67 antigen is immunohistochemical (IHC) analysis, and in spite of several data on Ki67 as a prognostic marker in early breast cancer, there are no standard operating procedures and accepted cut-offs to distinguish "Ki-67 high" from "Ki-67 low." For this reason, the role of Ki-67 in breast cancer management remains uncertain [65], and it was assumed that this marker is not ready for routine use.

The "International Ki-67 in Breast Cancer Working Group" established the IHC analysis as the more suitable method for measuring and monitoring tumor proliferation in standard pathology specimens and proposed guidelines for the analysis, reporting, and use of Ki-67 to reduce interlaboratory variability and improve interstudy comparability of Ki-67 results [70]:

- Type of biopsy: Core or whole section (whole section may give higher scores than core biopsy; when comparative scores are to be made, it is preferable to use the same type for both samples, e.g., in pre-surgical studies).
- Type of fixative: Neutral buffered formalin.
- Time of fixation: 8-72 hours.
- Means of storage: Tissue in paraffin bloc.
- Specific antibody: MIB1 or other antibodies against Ki67 antigen (MIB1 is the most widely validated antibody. SP6 antibody against Ki67 appears promising but insufficient data supports routine use at this time).
- Colorimetric detection system: Avidin–biotin immunoperoxidase or polymer detection.
- Method of reading:
    - Homogeneous staining: Count at least three randomly selected high-power (x40 objective) fields.
    - Heterogeneous staining:
- Hot spots: Assess the whole section, and record the overall average score.
- Gradient of increasing staining toward the tumor edge: Three fields should be scored at the periphery of the tumor.

Despite the lack of standardized procedures, in 13th St. Gallen Consensus Conference, the majority of the panelists voted that the threshold of ≥20% is clearly indicative of "high" Ki-67 status [66]. According to The American Society of Clinical Oncology (ASCO) Tumor Marker Guidelines Committee, the use of Ki-67 for prognosis in patients with newly identified breast cancer is not advised because of insufficient quality assurance [67]. Nonetheless, the clinical utility of Ki67 as a prognostic marker might be more apparent if it is considered within more tumor subgroups and/or as part of a multiparameter panel of biomarkers (estrogen receptor ER, progesterone receptor PgR, HER2) [68].

The immunopanel of ER, PgR, HER2, and Ki67 can segregate the luminal A and B subtypes: luminal breast cancers with Ki67 levels of at least 14% are defined as the luminal B subtype, which has a worse prognosis for both breast cancer recurrence and death; the tumors with Ki67 levels of less than 14% are luminal A [69]. A meta-analysis involving 12,155 patients also demonstrated that Ki-67 positivity confers a high risk of recurrence and a worse survival rate in patients with early breast cancer. Ki-67, is also used as an additional factor for decision-making on adjuvant treatment strategies.

References

[1] Senkus E, Kyriakides S, Penault-Llorca F, Poortmans P, Thompson A, Zackrisson S, Cardoso F. 2013. Primary breast cancer: ESMO Clinical Practice Guidelines for diagnosis, treatment and follow-up. *Ann. Oncol.* 24 Suppl 6: vi7-23.

[2] Narod SA. 2012. Breast cancer in young women. *Nat. Rev. Clin. Oncol.* 9: 460-70.

[3] Azim HA, Jr., Michiels S, Bedard PL, Singhal SK, Criscitiello C, Ignatiadis M, Haibe-Kains B, Piccart MJ, Sotiriou C, Loi S. 2012. Elucidating prognosis and biology of breast cancer arising in young women using gene expression profiling. Clin. Cancer Res. 18: 1341-51.

[4] Bharat A, Aft RL, Gao F, Margenthaler JA. 2009. Patient and tumor characteristics associated with increased mortality in young women (< or =40 years) with breast cancer. *J. Surg. Oncol.* 100: 248-51.

[5] Psyrri A, Burtness B. 2005. Pregnancy-associated breast cancer. *Cancer* J 11: 83-95.

[6] Rodriguez AO, Chew H, Cress R, Xing G, McElvy S, Danielsen B, Smith L. 2008. Evidence of poorer survival in pregnancy-associated breast cancer. *Obstet. Gynecol.* 112: 71-8.

[7] Moreira WB, Brandao EC, Soares AN, Lucena CE, Antunes CM. 2010. Prognosis for patients diagnosed with pregnancy-associated breast cancer: a paired case-control study. *Sao Paulo Med. J.* 128: 119-24.

[8] Azim HA, Jr., Botteri E, Renne G, Dell'orto P, Rotmensz N, Gentilini O, Sangalli C, Pruneri G, Di Nubila B, Locatelli M, Sotiriou C, Piccart M, Goldhirsch A, Viale G, Peccatori FA. 2012. The biological features and prognosis of breast cancer diagnosed during pregnancy: a case-control study. *Acta. Oncol.* 51: 653-61.

[9] Ishida T, Yokoe T, Kasumi F, Sakamoto G, Makita M, Tominaga T, Simozuma K, Enomoto K, Fujiwara K, Nanasawa T, et al. 1992. Clinicopathologic characteristics and prognosis of breast cancer patients associated with pregnancy and lactation: analysis of case-control study in Japan. *Jpn. J. Cancer* Res. 83: 1143-9.

[10] Guinee VF, Olsson H, Moller T, Hess KR, Taylor SH, Fahey T, Gladikov JV, van den Blink JW, Bonichon F, Dische S, et al. 1994. Effect of pregnancy on prognosis for young women with breast cancer. *Lancet* 343: 1587-9.

[11] Azim HA, Jr, Santoro L, Russell-Edu W, Pentheroudakis G, Pavlidis N, Peccatori FA. 2012. Prognosis of pregnancy-associated breast cancer: a meta-analysis of 30 studies. *Cancer Treat. Rev.* 38: 834-42.

[12] Berghofer A, Pischon T, Reinhold T, Apovian CM, Sharma AM, Willich SN. 2008. Obesity prevalence from a European perspective: a systematic review. *BMC Public Health* 8: 200.

[13] Protani M, Coory M, Martin JH. 2010. Effect of obesity on survival of women with breast cancer: systematic review and meta-analysis. *Breast Cancer Res. Treat.* 123: 627-35.

[14] Sparano JA, Wang M, Zhao F, Stearns V, Martino S, Ligibel JA, Perez EA, Saphner T, Wolff AC, Sledge GW, Jr., Wood WC, Fetting J, Davidson NE. 2012. Obesity at diagnosis is associated with inferior outcomes in hormone receptor-positive operable breast cancer. *Cancer* 118: 5937-46.

[15] Zhang S, Ivy JS, Payton FC, Diehl KM. 2010. Modeling the impact of comorbidity on breast cancer patient outcomes. *Health Care .Manag.* Sci. 13: 137-54.

[16] Girones R, Torregrosa D, Diaz-Beveridge R. 2010. Comorbidity, disability and geriatric syndromes in elderly breast cancer survivors. Results of a single - center experience. *Crit. Rev. Oncol. Hematol.* 73: 236-45.

[17] Satariano WA, Ragland DR. 1994. The effect of comorbidity on 3-year survival of women with primary breast cancer. *Ann. Intern. Med.* 120: 104-10.

[18] Houterman S, Janssen-Heijnen ML, Verheij CD, Louwman WJ, Vreugdenhil G, van der Sangen MJ, Coebergh JW. 2004. Comorbidity has negligible impact on treatment and complications but influences survival in breast cancer patients. *Br. J. Cancer* 90: 2332-7.

[19] Kaufman DW, Kelly JP, Rosenberg L, Anderson TE, Mitchell AA. 2002. Recent patterns of medication use in the ambulatory adult population of the United States: the Slone survey. *JAMA* 287: 337-44.

[20] Turner JP, Shakib S, Singhal N, Hogan-Doran J, Prowse R, Johns S, Bell JS. 2014. Prevalence and factors associated with polypharmacy in older people with cancer. *Support Care Cancer.*

[21] Hamaker ME, Seynaeve C, Wymenga AN, van Tinteren H, Nortier JW, Maartense E, de Graaf H, de Jongh FE, Braun JJ, Los M, Schrama JG, van Leeuwen-Stok AE, de Groot SM, Smorenburg CH. 2014. Baseline comprehensive geriatric assessment is associated with toxicity and survival in elderly metastatic breast cancer patients receiving single-agent chemotherapy: results from the OMEGA study of the Dutch Breast Cancer Trialists' Group. *Breast* 23: 81-7.

[22] Dawood S, Merajver SD, Viens P, Vermeulen PB, Swain SM, Buchholz TA, Dirix LY, Levine PH, Lucci A, Krishnamurthy S, Robertson FM, Woodward WA, Yang WT, Ueno NT, Cristofanilli M. 2011. International expert panel on inflammatory breast cancer: consensus statement for standardized diagnosis and treatment. *Ann. Oncol.* 22: 515-23.

[23] Shenkier T, Weir L, Levine M, Olivotto I, Whelan T, Reyno L. 2004. Clinical practice guidelines for the care and treatment of breast cancer: 15. Treatment for women with stage III or locally advanced breast cancer. *CMAJ* 170: 983-94.

[24] Bertucci F, Ueno NT, Finetti P, Vermeulen P, Lucci A, Robertson FM, Marsan M, Iwamoto T, Krishnamurthy S, Masuda H, Van Dam P, Woodward WA, Cristofanilli M, Reuben JM, Dirix L, Viens P, Symmans WF, Birnbaum D, Van Laere SJ. 2014. Gene expression profiles of inflammatory breast cancer: correlation with response to neoadjuvant chemotherapy and metastasis-free survival. *Ann. Oncol.* 25: 358-65

[25] Bates SE. 1991. Clinical applications of serum tumor markers. *Ann. Intern. Med.* 115: 623-38.

[26] Mirabelli P, Incoronato M. 2013. Usefulness of traditional serum biomarkers for management of breast cancer patients. *Biomed Res. Int.* 2013: 685641.

[27] Khatcheressian JL, Hurley P, Bantug E, Esserman LJ, Grunfeld E, Halberg F, Hantel A, Henry NL, Muss HB, Smith TJ, Vogel VG, Wolff AC, Somerfield MR, Davidson NE. 2013. Breast cancer follow-up and management after primary treatment: American Society of Clinical Oncology clinical practice guideline update. *J. Clin. Oncol.* 31: 961-5.

[28] Molina R, Barak V, van Dalen A, Duffy MJ, Einarsson R, Gion M, Goike H, Lamerz R, Nap M, Soletormos G, Stieber P. 2005. Tumor markers in breast cancer- European Group on Tumor Markers recommendations. *Tumour. Biol.* 26: 281-93.

[29] Evangelista L, Baretta Z, Vinante L, Cervino AR, Gregianin M, Ghiotto C, Saladini G, Sotti G. 2011. Tumour markers and FDG PET/CT for prediction of disease relapse in patients with breast cancer. Eur. J. Nucl. Med. Mol. Imaging 38: 293-301.

[30] Cardoso F, Harbeck N, Fallowfield L, Kyriakides S, Senkus E. 2012. Locally recurrent or metastatic breast cancer: ESMO Clinical Practice Guidelines for diagnosis, treatment and follow-up. *Ann. Oncol.* 23 Suppl 7: vii11-9.

[31] Siegel R, Naishadham D, Jemal A. Cancer statistics, 2013. *CA Cancer J. Clin.* (2013) 63:11–30. doi: 10.3322/caac.21166.

[32] Schairer C, Byrne C, Keyl PM, Brinton LA, Sturgeon SR, Hoover RN. Menopausal estrogen and estrogen-progestin replacement therapy and risk of breast cancer (United States). *Cancer Causes Control* (1994) 5:491–500. doi: 10.1007/BF01831376.

[33] Sprague BL, Trentham-Dietz A, Remington PL. The contribution of postmenopausal hormone use cessation to the declining incidence of breast cancer. *Cancer Causes Control* (2011) 22:125–34. doi: 10.1007/s10552-010-9682-7.

[34] Jemal A, Siegel R, Ward E, et al. Cancer statistics, 2007. *CA Cancer J. Clin.* 2007; 57(1):43–66.

[35] Jatoi I, Miller AB. Why is breast-cancer mortality declining? *Lancet Oncol.* 2003; 4(4):251–4.

[36] Cianfrocca M, Goldstein LJ. Prognostic and predictive factors in early-stage breast cancer. *Oncologist.* 2004; 9(6):606–16.

[37] Carter CL, Allen C, Henson DE. Relation of tumor size, lymph node status, and survival in 24,740 breast cancer cases. *Cancer.* 1989; 63(1):181–7.

[38] Harvey JN, Clark GM, Osborne CK, Allred DC. Estrogen receptor status by immunohistochemistry is superior to the ligand binding assay for predicting response to adjuvant endocrine therapy in breast cancer. *J. Clin. Oncol.* 1999; 17: 1474–1481.

[39] Clark GM. Prognostic and predictive factors. In: Harris JR, Lippman ME, Morrow M, Hellman S, eds. Diseases of the Breast. Philadelphia, Pa: Lippincott- Raven; 1996:461–485.

[40] Robert B Clarke. Steroid receptors and proliferation in the human breast. Steroids Volume 68, Issues 10–13, November 2003, Pages 789–794.

[41] Keen JC, Davidson NE. The biology of breast carcinoma. *Cancer.* 2003 Feb 1; 97(3 Suppl):825-33.

[42] Elledge RM, Allred DC: Clinical aspects of estrogen and progesterone receptors. In: Harris JR, Lippman ME, Morrow M, et al., (eds): Diseases of the Breast (ed 3). Philadelphia, PA, Lippincott Williams and Wilkins, 2004, pp 603-61.

[43] Albain K, Barlow W, O'Malley F, et al.: Concurrent (CAFT) versus sequential (CAF-T) chemohormonal therapy (cyclophosphamide, doxorubicin, 5-fluorouracil, tamoxifen) versus T alone for postmenopausal , node-positive, estrogen (ER) and/or progesterone (PgR) receptor-positive breast cancer: mature outcomes and new biologic correlates on phase III intergroup trial 0100 (SWOG-8814). [Abstract] *Breast Cancer Res .Treat.* 88 (Suppl 1): A-37, 2004.

[44] Issa J. Dahabreh, Helen Linardou, Fotios Siannis, George Fountzilas and Samuel Murray. Trastuzumab in the Adjuvant Treatment of Early-Stage Breast Cancer: A Systematic Review and Meta-Analysis of Randomized Controlled Trials. The Oncologist 2008, 13:620-630. doi: 10.1634/theoncologist.2008-0001.

[45] Patrick L. Fitzgibbons et al. Prognostic Factors in Breast Cancer. College of American Pathologists Consensus Statement 1999. *Arch. Pathol. Lab. Med..* 2000;124: 966–978.

[46] Prat A, Baselga J. The role of hormonal therapy in the management of hormonal-receptor-positive breast cancer with co-expression of HER2. Nat Clin Pract Oncol. 2008 Sep;5(9):531-42. doi: 10.1038/ncponc1179. Epub 2008 Jul 8.

[47] Early Breast Cancer Trialists' Collaborative Group (EBCTCG). Effects of chemotherapy and hormonal therapy for early breast cancer on recurrence and 15-year survival: an overview of the randomised trials. *Lancet* 2005 May 14-20;365(9472):1687-717.

[48] Allred DC, et al. Adjuvant tamoxifen reduces subsequent breast cancer in women with estrogen receptor-positive ductal carcinoma in situ: a study based on NSABP protocol B-24. *J. Clin. Oncol.* 2012 Apr 20;30 (12):1268-73. doi: 10.1200/JCO.2010.34.0141. Epub 2012 Mar 5.

[49] Fisher B, et al. Tamoxifen for the prevention of breast cancer: current status of the National Surgical Adjuvant Breast and Bowel Project P-1 study. *J. Natl. Cancer Inst.* 2005 Nov 16;97(22):1652-62.

[50] Buzdar AU, Vergote I, Sainsbury R. The impact of hormone receptor status on the clinical efficacy of the new-generation aromatase inhibitors: a review of data from first-line metastatic disease trials in postmenopausal women. *Breast J.* 2004 May-Jun;10(3):211-7.

[51] Dowsett M, et al. Retrospective analysis of time to recurrence in the ATAC trial according to hormone receptor status: an hypothesis-generating study. *J. Clin. Oncol.* 2005 Oct 20;23(30):7512-7.

[52] Viale G, et al. Prognostic and predictive value of centrally reviewed expression of estrogen and progesterone receptors in a randomized trial comparing letrozole and tamoxifen adjuvant therapy for postmenopausal early breast cancer: BIG 1-98. *J. Clin. Oncol.* 2007 Sep 1;25(25):3846-52. Epub 2007 Aug 6.

[53] Goss PE, et al. Efficacy of letrozole extended adjuvant therapy according to estrogen receptor and progesterone receptor status of the primary tumor: National Cancer Institute of Canada Clinical Trials Group MA.17. *J. Clin. Oncol.* 2007 May 20;25(15):2006-11. Epub 2007 Apr 23.

[54] Elizabeth Anderson. Progesterone receptors - animal models and cell signaling in breast cancer: The role of oestrogen and progesterone receptors in human mammary development and tumorigenesis. *Breast Cancer Res.* 2002, 4:197-201.

[55] Jacobsen BM, et al. Expression profiling of human breast cancers and gene regulation by progesterone receptors. *J. Mammary Gland. Biol. Neoplasia.* 2003 Jul;8(3):257-68.

[56] Schiff R, et al. Cross-talk between estrogen receptor and growth factor pathways as a molecular target for overcoming endocrine resistance. *Clin. Cancer Res.* 2004 Jan 1;10(1 Pt 2):331S-6S.

[57] Kampa M, Pelekanou V, Castanas E. Membrane-initiated steroid action in breast and prostate cancer. *Steroids.* 2008 Oct;73(9-10):953-60.

[58] Owens MA, Horten BC, Da Silva MM. HER2 amplification ratios by fluorescence in situ hybridization and correlation with immunohistochemistry in a cohort of 6556 breast cancer tissues. *Clin. Breast Cancer.* 2004 Apr; 5(1):63-9.

[59] Yaziji H, Goldstein LC, Barry TS, et al. HER-2 testing in breast cancer using parallel tissue-based methods. *JAMA.* 2004 Apr 28; 291(16):1972-7.

[60] Ariga R, Zarif A, Korasick J, Reddy V, Siziopikou K, Gattuso P. Correlation of her-2/neu gene amplification with other prognostic and predictive factors in female breast carcinoma. *Breast J.* (2005) 11:278–80.doi:10.1111/j. 1075-122x.2005.21463.x

[61] Maribeth Maher. *Current and Emerging Treatment Regimens for HER2-Positive Breast Cancer.* P&T® March 2014 Vol. 39 No. 3.

[62] Decensi A, Puntoni M, Pruneri G, Guerrieri Gonzaga A, Lazzeroni M, Serrano D, et al. Lapatinib activity in premalignant lesions and T cancer of the breast in a randomized, placebo-controlled pre surgical trial. *Cancer Prev Res* (Phila) (2011) 4:1181–9.doi:10. 1158/1940-6207. CAPR-10-0337.

[63] Antonio C. Wolff, et al. Hayes Steering Committee member Recommendations for Human Epidermal Growth Factor Receptor 2 Testing in Breast Cancer: American Society of Clinical Oncology/College of American Pathologists Clinical Practice Guideline Update. Published online ahead of print at www.jco.org on October 7, 2013. DOI: 10.1200/JCO.2013.50.9984.

[64] Gerdes J, Lemke H, Baisch H, Wacker HH, Schwab U, Stein H. Cell cycle analysis of a cell proliferation-associated human nuclear antigen defined by the monoclonal antibody Ki-67. *J. Immunol.* 1984;133(4):1710–1715.

[65] Yerushalmi R, Woods R, Ravdin PM, Hayes MM, Gelmon KA. Ki67 in breast cancer: prognostic and predictive potential. *Lancet Oncol.* 2010; 11(2):174–183.

[66] Goldhirsch, E. P. Winer, et al. Personalizing the treatment of women with early breast cancer: highlights of the St Gallen International Expert Consensus on the Primary Therapy of Early Breast Cancer 2013. *Annals of Oncology* 24: 2206–2223, 2013.

[67] Harris L, Fritsche H, Mennel R, Norton L, Ravdin P, Taube S, Somerfield MR, Hayes DF, Bast RC Jr (2007) American Society of Clinical Oncology 2007 update of recommendations for the use of tumor markers in breast cancer. *J. Clin. Oncol.* 25(33): 5287–5312.

[68] Cuzick J, Dowsett M, Wale C, et al. Prognostic value of a combined ER, PgR, Ki67, HER2 immunohistochemical (IHC4) score and the comparison with the GHI recurrence score—results from TransATAC. *Cancer Res.* 2009;69(suppl 24):503s.

[69] Cheang MC, Chia SK, Voduc D, Gao D, Leung S, Snider J. Ki67 index, HER2 status, and prognosis of patients with luminal B breast cancer. *J. Natl. Cancer Inst.* 2009; 101: 736–50.

[70] Dowsett M, Nielsen TO, A'Hern R, Bartlett J, Coombes RC, Cuzick J, Ellis M, Henry NL, Hugh JC, Lively T et al., (2011) Assessment of Ki67 in breast cancer: recommendations from the International Ki67 in Breast Cancer Working Group. *J. Natl. Cancer Inst.* 103:1656–1664.

[71] Lee RC, Feinbaum RL, Ambros V. The C. elegans heterochronic gene lin-4 encodes small RNAs with antisense complementarity to lin-14. *Cell.* 1993 Dec 3; 75(5):843-54.

[72] Wightman B, Ha I, Ruvkun G. Posttranscriptional regulation of the heterochronic gene lin-14 by lin-4 mediates temporal pattern formation in C. elegans. *Cell.* 1993 Dec 3; 75(5):855-62.

[73] Inui M, Martello G, Piccolo S. MicroRNA control of signal transduction. *Nat. Rev. Mol. Cell. Biol.* 2010 Apr; 11(4):252-63.

[74] Winter J, Jung S, Keller S, et al. Many roads to maturity: microRNA biogenesis pathways and their regulation. *Nat. Cell. Biol.* 2009 Mar; 11(3):228-34.

[75] Bartel DP. MicroRNAs: target recognition and regulatory functions. *Cell.* 2009 Jan 23; 136(2):215-33.

[76] Djuranovic S, Nahvi A, Green R. A parsimonious model for gene regulation by miRNAs. *Science.* 2011 Feb 4; 331(6017):550-3.

[77] O'Donnell KA, Wentzel EA, Zeller KI, et al. c-Myc-regulated microRNAs modulate E2F1 expression. *Nature.* 2005 Jun 9;435(7043):839-43

[78] Ma L, Young J, Prabhala H, et al. miR-9, a MYC/MYCN-activated microRNA, regulates E-cadherin and cancer metastasis. *Nat. Cell. Biol.* 2010 Mar; 12(3):247-56.

[79] Chang TC, Yu D, Lee YS, et al. Widespread microRNA repression by Myc contributes to tumorigenesis. *Nat. Genet.* 2008 Jan; 40(1):43-50.

[80] Calin GA, Dumitru CD, Shimizu M, et al. Frequent deletions and downregulation of micro-RNA genes miR15 and miR16 at 13q14 in chronic lymphocytic leukemia. *Proc. Natl. Acad. Sci. U S A.* 2002 Nov 26; 99(24):15524-9.

[81] Croce CM. Causes and consequences of microRNA dysregulation in cancer. *Nat. Rev. Genet.* 2009 Oct; 10(10):704-14.

[82] Lu J, Getz G, Miska EA, et al. MicroRNA expression profiles classify human cancers. *Nature.* 2005 Jun 9; 435(7043):834-8.

[83] Munker R, Calin GA. MicroRNA profiling in cancer. *Clin. Sci.* (Lond). 2011 Aug; 121(4):141-58.

[84] Volinia S, Calin GA, Liu CG, et al. MicroRNA expression signature of human solid tumors defines cancer gene targets. *Proc. Natl. Acad. Sci. U S A.* 2006 Feb 14; 103(7):2257-61.

[85] Calin GA, Croce CM. MicroRNA signatures in human cancers. *Nat. Rev. Cancer.* 2006 Nov;6 (11):857-66.

[86] Garzon R, Fabbri M, Cimmino A, et al. MicroRNA expression and function in cancer. *Trends Mol. Med.* 2006 Dec; 12(12):580-7.

[87] Murakami Y, Yasuda T, Saigo K, et al. Comprehensive analysis of microRNA expression patterns in hepatocellular carcinoma and non-tumorous tissues. *Oncogene.* 2006 Apr 20;25 (17):2537-45.

[88] Yanaihara N, Caplen N, Bowman E, et al. Unique microRNA molecular profiles in lung cancer diagnosis and prognosis. *Cancer Cell.* 2006 Mar;9 (3):189-98.

[89] Weber B, Stresemann C, Brueckner B, et al. Methylation of human microRNA genes in normal and neoplastic cells. *Cell. Cycle.* 2007 May 2;6(9):1001-5.

[90] Brueckner B, Stresemann C, Kuner R, et al. The human let-7a-3 locus contains an epigenetically regulated microRNA gene with oncogenic function. *Cancer Res.* 2007 Feb 15;67 (4):1419-23.

[91] Iorio MV, Visone R, Di Leva G, et al. MicroRNA signatures in human ovarian cancer. *Cancer Res.* 2007 Sep 15;67(18):8699-707.

[92] Jansson MD, Lund AH. MicroRNA and cancer. *Mol. Oncol.* 2012 Dec; 6(6):590-610.

[93] Bui TV, Mendell JT. Myc: Maestro of MicroRNAs. *Genes. Cancer.* 2010 Jun 1; 1(6):568-575.

[94] Kent OA, Chivukula RR, Mullendore M, et al. Repression of the miR-143/145 cluster by oncogenic Ras initiates a tumor-promoting feed-forward pathway. *Genes. Dev.* 2010 Dec 15;24(24):2754-9.

[95] Burk U, Schubert J, Wellner U, et al. A reciprocal repression between ZEB1 and members of the miR-200 family promotes EMT and invasion in cancer cells. *EMBO Rep.* 2008 Jun; 9(6):582-9.

[96] Chang TC, Wentzel EA, Kent OA, et al. Transactivation of miR-34a by p53 broadly influences gene expression and promotes apoptosis. *Mol. Cell.* 2007 Jun 8; 26(5):745-52.

[97] He L, He X, Lim LP, et al. A microRNA component of the p53 tumour suppressor network. *Nature.* 2007 Jun 28; 447(7148):1130-4.

[98] Hermeking H. MicroRNAs in the p53 network: micromanagement of tumour suppression. *Nat. Rev. Cancer.* 2012 Sep; 12(9):613-26.

[99] Bertos NR and Park M. Breast cancer — one term, many entities?. J. *Clin. Invest.* 2011;121(10):3789–3796.

[100] Iorio MV, Ferracin M, Liu CG, Veronese A, Spizzo R, Sabbioni S et al. MicroRNA gene expression deregulation in human breast cancer. *Cancer Res.,* 65 (2005 Aug 15), pp. 7065–7070.

[101] Zhang ZJ, Ma SL. miRNAs in breast cancer tumorigenesis (Review).*Oncol. Rep.* 2012 Apr; 27(4):903-10.

[102] Lv M, Zhu X, Chen W, Zhao J, Tang J. Searching for candidate microRNA biomarkers in detection of breast cancer: A meta-analysis. *Cancer Biomark.* 2013 Jan 1; 13(5):395-401.

[103] Ma L, Teruya-Feldstein J, Weinberg RA. Tumour invasion and metastasis initiated by microRNA-10b in breast cancer. *Nature* 449 (7163),682–688 (2007).

[104] Ma L, Young J, Prabhala H et al. miR-9, a MYC/MYCN-activated microRNA, regulates E-cadherin and cancer metastasis. *Nat. Cell Biol.* 12 (3),247–256 (2010).

[105] Tavazoie SF, Alarcon C, Oskarsson T et al. Endogenous human microRNAs that suppress breast cancer metastasis. *Nature* 451(7175),147–152 (2008).

[106] Valastyan S, Reinhardt F, Benaich N et al. A pleiotropically acting microRNA, miR-31, inhibits breast cancer metastasis. *Cell.* 137 (6),1032–1046 (2009).

[107] Buffa FM, Camps C, Winchester L et al. microRNA-associated progression pathways and potential therapeutic targets identified by integrated mRNA and microRNA expression profiling in breast cancer. *Cancer Res.*71 (17),5635–5645 (2011).

[108] Rothé F, Ignatiadis M, Chaboteaux C et al. Global microRNA expression profiling identifies miR-210 associated with tumor proliferation, invasion and poor clinical outcome in breast cancer. *PLoS ONE*6 (6),e20980 (2011).

[109] Foekens JA, Sieuwerts AM, Smid M et al. Four miRNAs associated with aggressiveness of lymph node-negative, estrogen receptor-positive human breast cancer. *Proc. Natl. Acad. Sci. USA*10 5(35),13021–13026 (2008).

[110] Camps C, Buffa FM, Colella S et al. hsa-miR-210 is induced by hypoxia and is an independent prognostic factor in breast cancer. Clin. Cancer Res.14(5),1340–1348 (2008).

[111] Healy NA, Heneghan HM, Miller N, Osborne CK, Schiff R, Kerin MJ. Systemic mirnas as potential biomarkers for malignancy. *Int. J. Cancer.* 2012 Nov 15;131(10):2215-22.

[112] Heneghan HM, Miller N, Lowery AJ, et al. Circulating microRNAs as novel minimally invasive biomarkers for breast cancer. *Ann. Surg.* 2010; 251: 499–505.

[113] Heneghan HM, Miller N, Kelly R, et al. Systemic miRNA-195 differentiates breast cancer from other malignancies and is a potential biomarker for detecting noninvasive and early stage disease. *Oncologist* 2010; 15: 673–82.

[114] Roth C, Rack B, Muller V, et al. Circulating microRNAs as blood-based markers for patients with primary and metastatic breast cancer. *Breast Cancer Res.* 2010; 12: R90.

[115] Wang F, Zheng Z, Guo J, et al. Correlation and quantitation of microRNA aberrant expression in tissues and sera from patients with breast tumor. *Gynecol. Oncol.* 2010; 119: 586–93.

[116] McShane LM, Altman DG, Sauerbrei W, Taube SE, Gion M, Clark GM. REporting recommendations for tumour MARKer prognostic studies (REMARK). *Br. J. Cancer* 93 (4),387–391 (2005).

[117] Smith B, Selby P, Southgate J, Pittman K, Bradley C and Blair GE Detection of melanoma cells in peripheral blood by means of reverse transcriptase and polymerase chain reaction. 1991 *Lancet* 338 1227–1229.

[118] Cristofanilli M, et al. Circulating tumor cells, disease progression, and survival in metastatic breast cancer. 2004 *New England Journal of Medicine* 321 781–79.

[119] Harris L, et al. American Society of Clinical Oncology 2007 update of recommendations for the use of tumor markers in breast cancer. 2007 J. *Clin. Oncol.* 25 5287–5312.

[120] Fehm T, et al. Methods for isolating circulating epithelial cells and criteria for their classification as carcinoma cells. 2005 *Cytotherapy* 7 171–185.

[121] Matro JM, Goldstein LJ. 2014. How do I follow patients with early breast cancer after completing adjuvant therapy. *Curr. Treat. Options Oncol.* 15: 63-78.

[122] Grunfeld E, Mant D, Yudkin P, Adewuyi-Dalton R, Cole D, Stewart J, Fitzpatrick R, Vessey M. 1996. Routine follow up of breast cancer in primary care: randomised trial. *BMJ* 313: 665-9.

[123] Grunfeld E, Levine MN, Julian JA, Coyle D, Szechtman B, Mirsky D, Verma S, Dent S, Sawka C, Pritchard KI, Ginsburg D, Wood M, Whelan T. 2006. Randomized trial of long-term follow-up for early-stage breast cancer: a comparison of family physician versus specialist care. *J. Clin. Oncol.* 24: 848-55.

[124] 1994. Impact of follow-up testing on survival and health-related quality of life in breast cancer patients. A multicenter randomized controlled trial. The GIVIO Investigators. *JAMA* 271: 1587-92.

[125] Pierce JP, Stefanick ML, Flatt SW, Natarajan L, Sternfeld B, Madlensky L, Al-Delaimy WK, Thomson CA, Kealey S, Hajek R, Parker BA, Newman VA, Caan B, Rock CL. 2007. Greater survival after breast cancer in physically active women with high vegetable-fruit intake regardless of obesity. *J. Clin. Oncol.* 25: 2345-51.

[126] Chlebowski RT, Blackburn GL, Thomson CA, Nixon DW, Shapiro A, Hoy MK, Goodman MT, Giuliano AE, Karanja N, McAndrew P, Hudis C, Butler J, Merkel D, Kristal A, Caan B, Michaelson R, Vinciguerra V, Del Prete S, Winkler M, Hall R, Simon M, Winters BL, Elashoff RM. 2006. Dietary fat reduction and breast cancer outcome: interim efficacy results from the Women's Intervention Nutrition Study. *J. Natl. Cancer Inst.* 98: 1767-76.

In: Prognostic and Predictive Response ... ISBN: 978-1-63463-545-5
Editors: V. Canzonieri and M. Berretta

Chapter 2

Colorectal Cancer: Prognostic and Predictive Response Therapy Factors

M. Berretta*[1,5*]*, G. Nasti*[2]*, V. Canzonieri*[3]*, M. Di Vita*[2]*,
***U. Tirelli*[1] *and C. De Divitiis*[4]**

[1]Department of Medical Oncology, CRO - National Cancer Institute, IRCCS Aviano, Italy

[2]Department of Surgery, University of Catania, Catania Italy

[3]Division of Pathology, CRO - National Cancer Institute, IRCCS Aviano, Italy

[4] Medical Oncology SUN of Naples and IRCCS Fondazione Pascale Napoli, Italy

[5]Euro-Mediterranean Institute of Science and Technology (IEMEST), Palermo, Italy

Abstract

Colorectal cancer (CRC) is the third most common cancer worldwide. Its prognosis is closely related to the stage of the disease at

* Correspondence to: Massimiliano Berretta, MD, Ph.D, Department of Medical Oncology, CRO Aviano - National Cancer Institute, Via F. Gallini 2 Aviano (PN) 33081 Italy, Phone +39 434 659724, Mobile +39 333 3914670, Fax +39 0434 659531, e-mail: mberretta@cro.it

the time of diagnosis. This is a review on the role of pathological classical factors, serum/clinical biomarkers and characteristics with prognostic and predictive response therapy value in the management of CRC. Clinical follow-up in CRC is of paramount importance in the correct approach to this disease. Moreover, molecular studies have recently widened the opportunity for testing new possible markers, but actually, only few markers can be recommended for practical use in clinic. In the next future the hope will be to have a complete panel of clinical biomarkers to use in every setting of CRC disease, and at the same time to receive information about prognostic significance by their expression and to be oriented in the choice of the adequate treatment.

Introduction

Over the past 30 years, the interest in clinical and molecular prognostic factors in metastatic colorectal cancer (mCRC) has grown.

This interest is even greater today with the advent of molecularly targeted agents, that have changed dramatically the treatment algorithms and survival for patients with mCRC.

CRC is one of the most commonly diagnosed cancers in the world and remains the second leading cause of death in United States.

Survival for patients with mCRC has improved dramatically over the past decade. In the mid 1990s, the median overall survival (OS) for patients with metastatic colon cancer treated with a 5-fluorouracil (5-FU)-based regimen was only about 12 months [1]. With the addition of irinotecan and oxaliplatin, OS increased to approximately 18 months [2-5], but it has really been the addition of biologic agents that led to a substantial jump in OS, approaching 30 months in some studies and significant advances have been made in the study of CRC, prognosis and outcome.

Despite the advances in dosing and scheduling of chemotherapy in both adjuvant and advanced settings, and a greater emphasis on early detection, for most patients the outlook still remains poor.

Molecular analyses have shown that the natural history of each CRCs differs. Cancers belonging to a particular pathologic stage may display significant clinical heterogeneity, which may reflect on the underlying molecular heterogeneity.

Individual patients with same stage tumours may have different long term prognosis and response to therapy. In addition, some prognostic variables are likely to be more important than others. This led to extensive research of other possible prognostic factors over the last eight decades, in attempt to improve identification of patients likely to have a poorer clinical outcome and therefore more likely to benefit from more aggressive treatment strategies.

Selection of the most beneficial treatment regimes in CRC remains a challenge and is hindered by the lack of well established markers correlating with survival or disease free survival (DFS) and markers predicting response to a particular therapy (prognostic and predictive markers, respectively).

Therefore, the information on which parameters influence prognosis would be valuable in the interpretation and design of clinical trials and also have implications for clinical decisions management in the palliative setting.

Clinical Prognostic Factors

Clinical trials, although using similar patient selection criteria, often display a surprising heterogeneity in survival rates [6], usually explained by differences in patient characteristics or prognostic factors. Patients entering randomised trials are typically stratified according to their performance status (PS), but in addition, other prognostic factors or their constellation may have the potential to determine the survival of patients to a greater extent than any promising antineoplastic agent or drug combination. A variety of clinical parameters such as PS [7], elevated lactate dehydrogenase, white blood cell (WBC) count [8], serum albumin [6], elevated liver transaminases [8], level of haemoglobin [9] or platelets, pathological grading [9] or localisation of the primary tumour [10], or tumour markers like carcinoembryonic antigen (CEA) [8] have been identified as prognostic markers in some studies that seldom included more than 400 patients. There is no consensus and general acceptance about the importance of various prognostic factors. Köhne's prognostic classification has been based on PS, alkaline phosphatase level, number of metastatic sites and WBCs count.

In a pooled analysis of source data from patients treated with FU for MCRC in 22 clinical trials, Köhne et al. divided patients into three prognostic groups (low, intermediate, and high risk) according to baseline factors: Eastern Cooperative Oncology Group (ECOG) PS, WBC count, alkaline phosphatase (ALP), and number of sites of metastatic disease. The low-risk patients had a median survival of 15 months, intermediate-risk patients had 11 months, and the high-risk patients had 6 months. Diaz et al. [11] proved the applicability of Köhne's classification in a limited number of patients treated with irinotecan- or oxaliplatin-based first-line chemotherapy. Sanoff et al. [12], analyzing the data from patients enrolled in the N9741 study, subsequently confirmed the validity of the score. ALP is a key prognostic factor as demonstrated in the GERCOR OPTIMOX 1 study [13], where patients with high levels of ALP (3-5 times the upper limit value) achieved significant shorter median progression-free and OS than patients with ALP ≤3 times the upper limit value.

Desot et. Al [14] suggested that the relevance of Köhne's classification is questionable. A simplified score could be validated by largest studies, based on WBCs count and PS.

Recently some reports have reported that the concomitant diagnosis of HIV-infection and CRC, represents an independent and poor prognostic factor in this particular setting of patients[15-18].

Conversely old age does not represent, after accurate evaluation (Comprehensive Geriatric Assessment), a poor prognostic factor [19-24].

The Peritoneal Involvement

The peritoneal involvement is an important independent pathological prognostic parameter and may supersede other parameters currently used in colonic cancer prognosis.

It is more frequently seen in colon cancer patients than among those with rectal cancer, because the cancer cells are more likely to shed into the peritoneal cavity following the serosal penetration. These patients occasionally present with ascites and weight loss before the discovery of the colorectal primary. The prognosis of these patients is dismal. In patients with stage IV, the presence of peritoneal carcinomatosis is associated with a significant reduction in survival, from 18.1 months to 6.7 months [25]. Treatment has traditionally been palliative with systemic chemotherapy when diagnosis is established before surgery.

The presence of peritoneal metastases (PM) from CRC has been considered a terminal stage of disease, and patients have been offered the best supportive care and/or systemic chemotherapy with or without palliative surgery. Surgery or chemotherapy alone have not improve the patients' survival resulting in a median survival of 5–7 months. Over the past two decades, a new therapeutic alternative approach based on the combination of surgery with chemotherapy has been developed as a treatment of PM.

Peritoneal carcinomatosis is often associated with metastatic disease, although the peritoneal cavity appears to be the only site of the disease in about 25% of patients. Several groups have advocated the use of cytoreductive surgery and hyperthermic intraperitoneal chemotherapy (HIPEC) as a means of improving survival in these patients [26]. This treatment, however, is associated with significant morbidity and mortality. A randomized trial from the Netherlands comparing cytoreduction surgery plus HIPEC with systemic chemotherapy plus palliative surgery have found that patients in the former group exhibit a statistically significant improvement in median survival (22.3 months vs. 12.6 months). Cytoreductive surgery plus HIPEC seems to be a viable option for the treatment of peritoneal carcinomatosis. Patient selection for these aggressive procedures remains a major issue, given the substantial morbidity and mortality associated with them. Prognosis in these patients depends on the extent of carcinomatosis, the ability to achieve a complete cytoreduction and the tumour biology. Da eliminare completamente.

Sites of Metastatic Disease

Regarding the sites of metastatic disease, Assersohn et al., (reference) have found that the most important positive predictor for OS was the presence of liver metastases. In their study, the authors have shown that the presence of liver metastases was a better predictor for response that both PS and number of sites of metastatic disease. Increased of CEA level, decreased of albumin level, poor PS, PM, and bolus of 5-Fu treatment were the predictive indicators of poor response rate and increased mortality in patients treated with 5Fu for metastatic CRC.

The Predictive Value of Early Metabolic PET/CT Response

With the availability of many new drugs and molecular targeted therapies, the need for the medical oncologist to obtain information that can somehow predict the effectiveness of a treatment or giving information on a possible response to the same has become stronger.

Today, more than traditional radiology, the nuclear medicine techniques such as 18 F-FDG PET, seem to meet part of these new needs. Especially, Lastoria et al. [27] have shown how early changes in tumour metabolism measured by PET/CT with 18 F–FDG could predict the efficacy of treatment better than standard RECIST response. In their experience, the authors analyzed 33 patient with resectable liver metastases from CRC, within a phase 2 trial of preoperative FOLFIRI plus bevacizumab. PET/CT evaluations have been performed before and after one cycle of FOLFIRI plus bevacizumab, concluding that PET/CT response was significantly predictive of long term outcomes during preoperative treatment of patients with resectable liver metastases from CRC. Clearly, larger studies are needed to confirm these results.

Recently, Celik et al. [28] have found that level of TNF-related apoptosis-inducing-ligand and CXCL8 correlate with 2-[18F] Fluoro-2-deoxy-D-glucose uptake in 29 patients with mCRC treated with bevacizumab. They have evaluated the changes and correlations of TRAIL (TNF-related apoptosis-inducing-ligand) and CXCL8 (IL8) prior to treatment and three months following therapy as well as the corresponding PET/CT. Generally, sTRAIL values were increased during therapy, while a decrease was observed for CXCL8. Correlation analysis has been applied to the data and revealed significant correlations for the SUVmax in the primary tumour prior to treatment and CXCL8 prior to therapy ($p=0.0303$). Furthermore, significant correlations have been observed for the SUVmax and sTRAIL ($p=0.0237$) as well as CXCL8 ($p=0.0002$) three months after treatment initiation. CXCL8 prior to treatment has been also correlated with the SUV three months after onset of treatment ($p=0.0072$). Also, they have noted a significant correlation for one combination of two variables, the SUVmax in the metastases and CXCL8 prior to treatment ($p=0.0175$). These results are supported when grouping the SUVmax in the metastases following treatment into two groups with SUVmax <5 and SUVmax>5. Therefore, this study have provided evidence that proteomics patterns of sTRAIL and CXCL8 predict tumour response and survival in MCRC patients treated with bevacizumab and within a high concordance of FDG-PET/CT findings.

Prognostic Serum Markers

The role of CEA as prognostic factor in mCRC is unclear. High levels of serum CEA on diagnosis has been associated with a worse poor prognosis in some studies, while some authors have found no significant correlation between CEA and prognosis. For instance, Webb et al., (reference), showed that CEA, Ca 125 and BHCG (>40mIU/L only) are correlated with poor prognosis on univariate and multivariate analyses; serum AFP and Ca 19.9 levels instead, had no prognostic value.

Selcukbiricik et al., [29] aimed to determine the prognostic role of initial CEA and CA 19-9 values in mCRC. The Authors, between 2000 and 2010, have analyzed a total of 215 patients with mCRC who were treated and followed up in Turkey. The initial CEA and CA19-9 values were determined. K-ras mutation analysis was performed using quantitative PCR evaluation of the DNA from the tumour tissues. (RISULTATI?)

Beak et al., [30] assessed the relationship between serpin B5 and CEA expression in CRC. Serpin B5 is a candidate tumour suppressor, but its oncogenic activity has also been reported. Its function may be affected by protein interactions. They analyzed the clinic-pathological significance of serpin B5 expression in patients with CRC. Tissue expression of serpin B5 in 377 patients with CRC was significantly associated with serum CEA, histological grade, stage, lymph node metastasis, lymphatic and perineural invasion, and infiltrative border. Strong expression of serpin B5 was also associated with a reduced DFS ($p = 0.001$) and OS ($p = 0.017$). Together, these findings describe a relationship between serpin B5 and CEA expression in CRC. Strong expression of serpin B5 has been associated with a worse prognosis in patients with CRC and its expression may correlate with CEA levels in CRC.

K-ras mutations have been detected in 99 of the patients (46%). K-ras has been found to be wild type in 116 patients (54%). Significant differences have been detected between the K-ras wild-type and mutant groups with respect to age and the initial serum CEA levels. The median OS time and 3-year OS rate for patients with a high initial CEA level (>5 ng/mL) have been significantly shorter than those of patients with a low initial CEA level (<5 ng/mL) (50.5 months and 61.8% vs. 78.6 months and 79.1%, $p=0.014$). Multivariate analysis have indicated that stage at the time of diagnosis ($p<0.001$) and low initial serum CEA level ($p=0.037$) are independent prognostic factors of OS. For K-ras mutant patients, the stage at diagnosis ($p=0.017$), low initial serum CEA level ($p=0.001$), and low initial serum CA 19-9 level have been found to be independent prognostic indicators of OS. Thus, they have demonstrated for the first time that the presence of a K-ras mutation correlates with high initial CEA and CA 19-9 levels in patients with mCRC.

Serum CA19-9 (carbohydrate antigen 19-9) level has been reported as a factor predictive of survival in patients with colorectal cancer. A few articles have reported that patients with mCRC who have normal (< or =37 U/mL) serum CA19-9 levels survived significantly longer than those with higher serum CA19-9 levels. However, these reports are contradictory and lack definite conclusions.

Wang et al. [31] have found that serum CA19-9 level is the most significant and independent prognostic indicator of patients with mCRC and they have recommended that stratification for further clinical trials for patients with mCRC should be carried out according to serum CA19-9 levels.

Prognostic Tissue Factors

Macro-Microscopic Characteristics

Most CRC are adenocarcinomas of which mucinous and signet ring adenocarcinoma constitute approximately 10%, with signet ring carcinoma comprising 1–2.4%. Mucinous cancers are defined histologically by the presence of abundant extracellular mucin, with more than 50% of the tumour mass being mucinous. Signet ring cancers have intracellular mucin pushing the nucleus to one side.

The signet ring cell type of adenocarcinoma and undifferentiated carcinoma are subtypes of colonic carcinoma that have been demonstrated by multivariate analysis to have an independent adverse impact on prognosis. These tumours are respectively assigned grade 3/4 (poorly differentiated) and grade 4/4 (undifferentiated). Therefore, both of these types of tumour are considered high grade and associated with an unfavourable prognosis. Mucinous histology of metastatic CRC has been associated with poor prognosis [32], however this has never been assessed in large well-defined study populations treated with the currently available systemic agents.

Yamaguchi et al. [33] have confirmed that patients with metastatic mucinous CRC have distinct clinico-pathological features and poor response to chemotherapy and targeted agents. The strong negative prognostic value of mucinous histology (?) warrants the use of this pathological feature as a stratification factor for clinical trials in metastatic CRC. The mCRC extension into an adjacent structure or organ and involvement of the parietal peritoneum (serosal involvement), has been demonstrated to have independent adverse prognostic significance.

Patients with pT4 tumours penetrating the visceral peritoneum have a shorter median survival time after surgical resection compared to patients with pT3 tumours that lack serosal involvement, in either the presence or absence of distal metastases. Based on this adverse effect on outcome, it has been suggested that tumours in the T4 category be further classified as T4a (tumours involving the visceral peritoneum) and T4b (tumours invading adjacent structures or organs). In summary pathological macro-microscopic prognostic factors rely on:

1. Characteristic of the primary tumor: gross appearance (Figure 1 A e B), anatomic extent of disease, level of circumferential involvement, bowel obstruction, perforation, pattern of invasion, grade of differentiation.
2. Vascular invasion: extramural venous involvement, lymphatic or perineural space involvement (Figure 2), reactive changes in regional lymph nodes.
3. Host response: angiogenensis, local inflammation, local desmoplastic reaction;
4. Post surgical factors: distance between resection margins and tumor; presence of residual tumor.

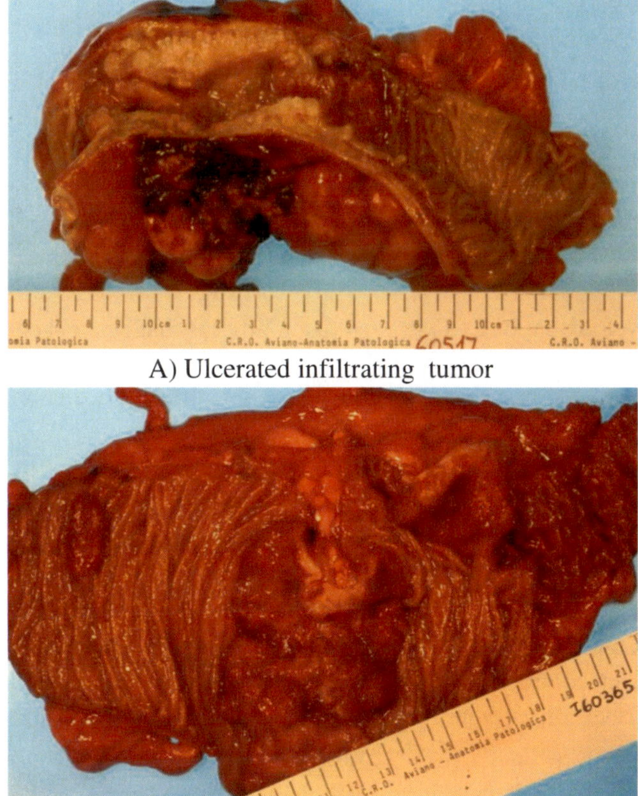

A) Ulcerated infiltrating tumor

B) Polypoid tumors: adenoma on the right upper corner and a polypoid cancer on the centre

Figure 1. Different gross appearances of colon cancer.

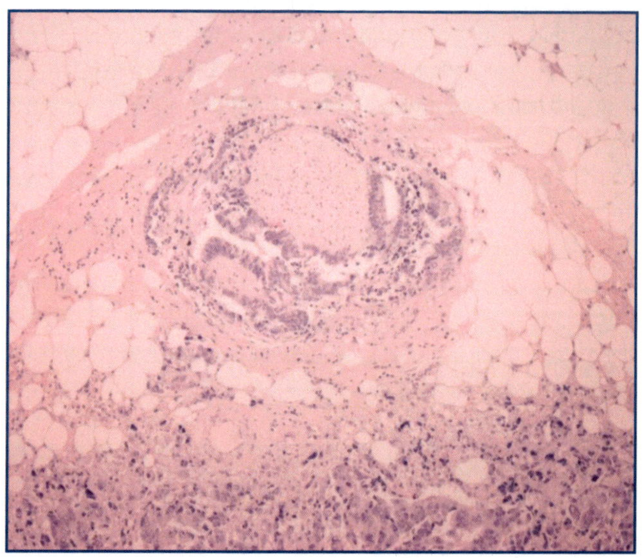

Figure 2. Istological documentation of perineural invasion in colon cancer (adverse prognosis).

Molecular Prognostic and Predictive Markers

The development of CRC is a multistep process that occurs because of the accumulation of several genetic alterations, including chromosomal abnormalities, gene mutations, and epigenetic modifications involving several genes that regulate proliferation, differentiation, apoptosis, and angiogenesis.

Molecular analyses have shown that the natural history of all CRCs is not the same [34]. Cancers belonging to a particular pathologic stage may display significant clinical heterogeneity, which may reflect an underlying molecular heterogeneity.

Among the various genetic alterations, the epidermal growth factor receptor (EGFR) is an important molecular target for mCRC treatment. EGFR is activated in colorectal carcinogenesis by the binding of a ligand on the extracellular part of it (Figure 3). The autophosphorylation of the intracellular tyrosine kinase domain of the EGFR activates downstream signalling pathways, including the Ras/raf/mitogen-activated protein kinase pathway, the phosphatidylinositol 3-kinase/Akt pathway, and the signal transduction and activator of transcription pathway, which interfere with apoptosis, cell proliferation, angiogenesis, and the metastatic process.

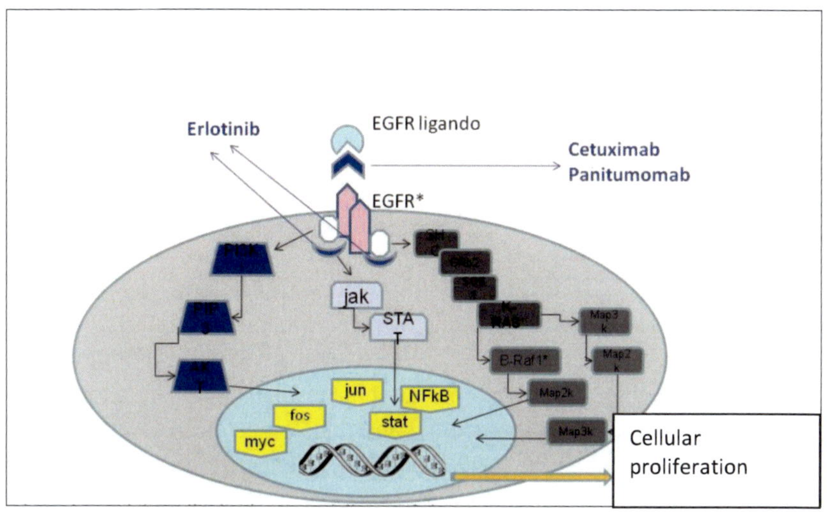

Figure 3. EGFR pathways.

EGFR, also known as HER1 or ErbB, is a 170-kD receptor tyrosine kinase and belongs to the ErbB receptor family. There are four members in the ErbB receptor family: ErbB1 (EGFR, HER1), ErbB2 (HER2/neu), ErbB3 (HER3), and ErbB4 (HER4). The binding of several specific ligands, such as EGF, TGF-, or amphiregulin, results in the dimerization of EGFR and subsequent phosphorylation of several tyrosine residues [35, 36].

These phosphorylated tyrosines serve as binding sites for several signal transducers that initiate multiple signaling pathways, including the Ras/Raf/MAP/MEK/ERK and/or PTEN/PI3K/Akt pathways.

Although EGFR plays important roles in cell differentiation and proliferation in normal cells, the activation of EGFR signalling is frequently observed in CRC cells, where it results in cell proliferation, migration and metastasis, evasion of apoptosis, or angiogenesis. Approximately 35% CRC tissues carry a mutation at codon 12 or 13 of *KRAS* that leads to the constitutive activation of EGFR downstream pathways [37–41].

Information on the *KRAS/NRAS/ BRAF* genotype is also extremely useful when selecting systemic chemotherapy for advanced and recurrent patients with CRC, helping identify patients with poor prognoses. *KRAS, NRAS* and *BRAF* are currently under focus as potential prognostic and predictive biomarkers in patients with metastatic diseases treated with anti-EGFR monoclonal antibodies (mAb), such as cetuximab and panitumumab [42-46].

Several retrospective analyses revealed that cetuximab treatment is ineffective in patients with *KRAS* mutations, thereby suggesting that the *KRAS* genotype is a useful predictive biomarker for cetuximab or panitumumab therapy in CRC. It has also been suggested that wild-type *BRAF* is required for a successful response to panitumumab or cetuximab therapies in patients with mCRC. However, the prognostic relevance of the KRAS genotype in CRC remains controversial despite several multi-institutional investigations since the 1990s [46-50].

The activation of EGFR signalling, such as Ras/Raf/MAP/ MEK/ERK and/or PTEN/PI3K/Akt pathways, constitutes a key step in tumourigenesis and tumour progression of CRC [51]. Two predominant EGFR inhibitors have been developed including monoclonal antibodies that target the extracellular domain of EGFR and small molecule TKIs that target the receptor catalytic domain of EGFR. Although both classes of agents show clear antitumor activity, only the anti-EGFR mAb has been approved for clinical use in the treatment of patients with metastatic CRC. Because the predictive value of alterations in EGFR expression level is unclear in the use of anti-EGFR mAb, the focus has shifted to alterations of key signalling pathways downstream of EGFR. In particular, *KRAS* and *BRAF* mutations have been studied as the activating mechanisms of the EGFR signalling pathway. Screening for *KRAS/BRAF* genotype is extremely important for identifying patients with shorter survival in response to systemic chemotherapy, regardless of the use of anti-EGFR mAb, and for predicting patients who would benefit from anti-EGFR mAb therapy. Therefore, the significance of *KRAS/BRAF* mutations as prognostic and/or predictive biomarkers in patients with CRC should be considered while selecting a method for *KRAS* genotyping. *KRAS* mutations were observed in approximately 35% patients with CRC, of which 25% patients had mutations at codon 12 and 10% patients had mutations at codon 13. The *KRAS* genotype is a useful predictive biomarker for patients with metastatic CRC treated with anti-EGFR mAb. Several studies have showed the possibility that *KRAS13* may have a specific phenotype that is different from other *KRAS* genotypes. Therefore, differences in *KRAS* mutations at codons 12 and 13 may result in different biological, biochemical, and functional consequences and clinical features, which may also influence the prognosis of CRC. In fact, a lot of retrospective analyses have suggested that *KRAS* mutations at codon 13, particularly *KRAS* p.G13D, as well as *BRAF* mutations are prognostic factors. Also, a study (reference?) showed that patients with *KRAS* p.G13D, but not other mutations, may experience a survival benefit from treatment with cetuximab plus chemotherapy.

In particular, Tejpar et al., [52] have investigated the associations between tumour *KRAS* mutation status (wild-type, G13D, G12V, or other mutations) and progression-free survival (PFS), survival and response in pooled data from 1,378 evaluable patients from the CRYSTAL and OPUS studies. Significant variations in treatment effects have been found for tumour response (*P*=0.005) and PFS (*P*=0.046) in patients with G13D-mutant tumours versus all other mutations (including G12V). Within *KRAS* mutation subgroups, cetuximab plus chemotherapy versus chemotherapy alone has significantly improved PFS (median, 7.4 vs. 6.0 months; hazard ratio [HR], 0.47; *P*=0.039) and tumour response (40.5% vs. 22.0%; odds ratio, 3.38; *P*=0.042) but not survival (median, 15.4 vs.14.7 months; HR, 0.89; *P*=0.68) in patients with G13D-mutant tumours. Patients with G12V and other mutations have not benefit from this treatment combination. Patients with *KRAS* G13D–mutated tumours receiving chemotherapy alone have experienced worse outcomes (response, 22.0% vs. 43.2%; odds ratio, 0.40; *P*=0.032) than those with other mutations. Effects were similar in the separate CRYSTAL and OPUS studies. The authors have concluded that the addition of cetuximab to first-line chemotherapy confers a benefit to patients with *KRAS* G13D–mutant tumours. These findings are also suggestive that patients with CRC having *KRAS* mutations constitute a heterogeneous population. Since the prognostic and/or predictive role of *KRAS13* mutations continues to remain controversial, further prospective clinical investigations are warranted. Also, KRAS wild-type status is an imperfect predictor of sensitivity to anti-EGFR monoclonal antibodies in colorectal cancer (CRC), motivating efforts to identify novel molecular aberrations driving RAS. The identification of *KRAS* mutations as markers of resistance to epidermal growth factor receptor (EGFR) inhibitors has paved the way to the interrogation of numerous other markers of resistance to anti-EGFR therapy, such as *NRAS*, *BRAF*, and PI3KCA mutations. Other genomic and protein expression alterations have been recently identified as potential targets of treatment or as markers of chemotherapy or targeted-therapy resistance, including ERCC1 expression, c-Met expression, PTEN expression, HER2 amplification, HER3 expression, and rare *KRAS* mutations. As the number of distinct validated intra-tumour genomic assays increases, numerous molecular assays will need to be compiled into one multigene panel assay. Several companies and academic centres are now offering multigene assays to patients with mCRC and other solid tumours.

Mutations in *KRAS* account for about 85% of all *RAS* mutations in human tumours, *NRAS* for about 15%, and *HRAS* for less than 1%. Each particular *RAS* gene mutation seems to be tumour specific; colonic, i.e., pancreatic and lung cancers have high frequencies of *KRAS* mutations. Nevertheless, there are only a few reports on *NRAS* mutations in colorectal cancer and none of these studies have correlated *RAS* mutations with other molecular events. Natsumi Irahara, et al. [51] have developed and validated a pyroseqencing assay to detect *NRAS* mutations at codons12, 13 and 61 and, utilizing a collection of 225 colorectal cancers from two prospective cohort studies, the authors have examined the relationship between *NRAS* mutations, clinical outcome, and other molecular features, including mutation of *KRAS*, *BRAF*, and *PIK3CA*, microsatellite instability (MSI), and the CpG island methylator phenotype (CIMP). Finally, they have examined whether *NRAS* mutation is associated with patient survival or prognosis. *NRAS* mutations have been detected in 5 (2.2%) of the 225 colorectal cancers and tended to occur in left-sided cancers arising in women, but have not appear to be associated with any of the molecular features that have been examined [51].

Several researches have suggested that tumours harbouring *BRAF* mutations have distinct clinic-pathological features compared with tumours harbouring *KRAS* mutations. Souglakos and associates have demonstrated that *BRAF* mutations in primary colorectal cancer mark patients with poor prognosis regardless of specific treatment regimen[53]. Patients with *BRAF* mutation have had significantly higher probability of disease progression (P<0.0001) or death (P<0.0001) with any treatment regimen. The *BRAF* V600E mutation has predicted independently early relapse on first-line therapy and death. It has been deduced that *BRAF* mutation does not simply substitute for *KRAS* activation in a linear signalling pathway but probably confers distinct impact on prognosis. It also has suggested that *KRAS* mutation may bypass aberrant EGFR signalling. In the PETACC-3 study which has included stage II and stage III cancer patients, *BRAF* tumour mutation has been found in 7.9% of cases and there has been no significant variability with tumour stage. In a multivariate analysis, *BRAF* mutation has been significantly associated with female sex, and has been highly significantly associated with right-sided tumours, older age, high grade, and MSI-high tumours. In univariate and multivariate analysis *BRAF* mutation has been not prognostic for relapse free survival but has been prognostic for OS, particularly in patients with MSI-L MSS tumours.

In the 2009 study by Souglakos et al., [53], patients with *BRAF* mutant tumours treated with cetuximab have also had lower progression free survival compared with those with *BRAF* wild type (0 vs. 17%), a finding which could partly explain resistance to anti EGFR targeted therapy in a subset of patients with tumours harbouring *KRAS* wild type. This is in keeping with an earlier study by Di Nicolantonio and colleagues [54], where the response to panitumumab or cetuximab has been found to be impeded by the presence of *BRAF* V600E mutation and restored (in a cellular model of CRC cells) by *BRAF* inhibitor sorafenib [55]. The authors have suggested that this experimental observation should encourage conceiving clinical trials using multiple therapies with EGFR and *BRAF*/MAPK inhibitors, considering that cetuximab, panitumumab, and sorafenib are already approved for clinical use.

Furthermore, *BRAF* mutations are significant negative prognostic biomarkers in patients with recurrent CRC across all disease stages. Besides, the prognostic value of *BRAF* mutations has been confirmed in patients with CRC treated with specific chemotherapy regimens in clinical trials evaluating a combination of cetuximab with chemotherapy. However, whether *BRAF* mutations are negative predictive biomarkers for anti-EGFR mAb has not been ascertained, because the controlled study, which directly compared the efficacy of adding anti-EGFR mAb to chemotherapy with that of chemotherapy alone, is lacking in a small population with *BRAF* mutations. The application of novel strategies targeting *BRAF* kinase is assured for the treatment of patients with CRC with *BRAF* mutations to improve their poor survival. However, clinical data suggest that the Ras/Raf/ERK pathway is insufficient for completely predicting the response to anti-EGFR mAbs. Thus, other factors, such as PIK3CA/PTEN deregulation and/or the expression status of epiregulin or amphiregulin, should also be studied on as possible predictive biomarkers for anti-EGFR mAb.

In line with these new evidence, Douillard et al. [56] have suggested that mutations in exons 3 and 4 *KRAS* and exons 2, 3 and 4 of *NRAS* represent factors of possible resistance to panitumumab. In particular, the population of patients with mCRC defined as “all ras wild type”, have presented in the PRIME study a significant advantage in survival: OS was 26.0 months in the panitumumab-FOLFOX4 group vs. 20.2 months in the FOLFOX4-alone group (hazard ratio for death, 0.78; 95% CI, 0.62 to 0.99; P=0.04) with the use of panitumumab in combination with FOLFOX compared to chemotherapy alone. Also, the analysis of the survival data has shown a detrimental effect of this combination in the population of patients "all mutated RAS". Finally, the PRIME study has confirmed the strong negative prognostic role of *BRAF* mutations, although these have not shown a clear predictive effect related to anti EGRF therapies.

PI3KCA mutation and PTEN deletion are two promising biomarkers that may predict resistance to anti EGFR therapy (e.g., cetuximab or panitumumab). Phosphatase and tensin homologue deleted on chromosome 10

(PTEN) negatively regulates the phosphoinositide-3-kinase (PI3K) signalling pathway. In colorectal cancer (CRC), observed frequencies of loss of PTEN expression, concordant expression in primary tumours and metastases, and the association of PTEN status with outcome vary markedly by detection method. Atreya et al., [57], determined the degree to which PTEN expression is consistent in 70 matched human CRC primaries and CRC primaries and liver metastases using a validated immune-histochemistry assay. Loss of PTEN expression in 12.3% of assessable CRC primaries and 10.3% of assessable liver metastases has been found. PTEN expression (positive or negative) was concordant in 98% of matched colorectal primaries and liver metastases. Next PTEN status has been related to mutations in RAS and PI3K pathway genes (*KRAS*, *NRAS*, *BRAF* , and PIK3CA) and to OS. PTEN expression was not significantly associated with the presence or absence of mutations in RAS or PI3K pathway genes. The median OS of patients whose tumours did not express PTEN was 9 months, compared to 49 months for patients whose tumours have expressed PTEN (HR=6.25, 95% confidence intervals (CI) (1.98, 15.42, P=0.0017). The association of absent PTEN expression with increased risk of death remained significant in multivariate analysis (HR=6.31, 95% CI (2.03, 17.93), P = 0.0023). In summary, PTEN expression has been consistent in matched CRC primaries and in liver metastases. Therefore, future investigations of PTEN in mCRC can use primary tumour tissue. In patients with liver-only metastases, loss of PTEN expression predicted poor OS. The authors have observed concordant PTEN expression in 98% of CRC primary and liver metastasis pairs using a validated immunohistochemistry assay. Consistent PTEN expression at both disease sites is significative because tumour tissue is usually available from CRC primaries but not metastases. Loss of PTEN expression is associated with poor survival of CRC patients with liver-only metastases.

Currently, conflicting information exists regarding Her-2 over-expression and its clinic-pathological implications in colorectal cancer (CRC). Lim SW et al., [58], have determined Her-2 over-expression in both serum and tumour tissue of 95 CRC patients and 60 healthy controls by chemiluminescent immunoassay and immune-histochemical staining. The results have been confirmed using fluorescent in situ hybridization. Clinico-pathological parameters have been analyzed according to Her-2 expression status. The authors have found that serum Her-2 levels were not significantly associated with prognostic parameters, concluding that Her-2 expression analysis of CRC tissue, but not in serum, acts as a significant independent worse prognostic factor. Then, the assessment of Her-2 expression status may be valuable for the targeted therapeutic management of CRC.

Among patients with CRC *KRAS* and *BRAF* are important biomarkers, although their role in patients undergoing surgical therapy for liver metastases remains unknown. Karagkounis et al. [59] have examined the incidence and prognostic significance of *KRAS* and *BRAF* mutations in patients undergoing surgery for colorectal liver metastases between 2003 and 2008. They have found *KRAS* mutations in approximately one third of patients, and *BFAF* mutations in only 2% of the patients examined. *KRAS* status have been resulted as an independent predictor of overall and recurrence-free survival.

Therefore, their experience has indicated that molecular biomarkers such as *KRAS* may help to refine the prognostic assessment of patients undergoing surgical therapy for colorectal liver metastases.

Clinical Follow-up

Periodic evaluations following the treatment of colon cancer, may lead to an earlier identification and management of recurrent disease [60]. After curative-intent surgery and adjuvant chemotherapy, if administered, post-treatment surveillance of patients with CRC is performed to evaluate possible therapeutic complications, discover any recurrence that is potentially resectable for cure, and identify new metachronous neoplasms at a pre-invasive stage. An analysis of data from 20.898 patients enrolled in 18 large, adjuvant, colon cancer, randomized trials has shown that 80% of recurrences occurred in the first 3 years after surgical resection of the primary tumor [61], and a recent study has found that 95% of recurrences occurred in the first 5 years [62].

Advances of more intensive follow-up of patients with stage II and/or stage III disease have been shown prospectively in several prior studies [63-65] and in 3 meta-analyses of randomized controlled trials designed to compare low-and high-intensity programs of surveillance [65-69]. Intensive postoperative surveillance has also been suggested to be of benefit to patients with stage I and IIA disease [70].

Furthermore, a population-based report indicates increased rates of respectability and survival in patients treated for local recurrence and distant metastases of CRC in more recent years, thereby providing support for more intensive post-treatment follow-up in these patients [71]. Results from a recent randomized controlled trial of 1202 patients with resected stage I to III disease showed that intensive surveillance imaging or CEA screening have resulted in an increased rate of curative-intent surgical treatment compared with a smaller follow-up group receiving testing only if symptoms occurred, but no advantage has been seen in the CEA and CT combination arm (2.3% in the minimum follow-up group, 6.7% in the CEA group, 8% in the CT group, and 6.6% in the CEA plus CT group) [72]. In this study, no mortality benefit to regular monitoring with CEA, CT, or both has been observed compared with minimum follow-up (death rate, 18.2% vs. 15.9%; difference, 2.3%; 95% CI, -2.6% to 7.1%). The authors have concluded that any strategy of surveillance is unlikely to provide a large survival advantage over a symptom-based approach.

For patients with stage I disease, the panel believes that a less intensive surveillance schedule is appropriate because of the low risk of recurrence and the harms associated with repeated CT scans, psychological stress associated with surveillance visits and scans, and risks from following up false-positive results. Therefore, for patients with stage I disease, the panel recommends colonoscopy at 1 year. Repeat colonoscopy is recommended at 3 years, and then every 5 years thereafter, unless advanced adenoma (villous polyp, polyp >1 cm, or high-grade dysplasia) is found. In this case, colonoscopy should be repeated in 1 year [73].

The following panel recommendations for post-treatment surveillance pertain to patients with stage II/III disease who have undergone successful treatment (i.e., no known residual disease). History and physical examination should be given every 3 to 6 months for 2 years, and then every 6 months for a total of 5 years. A CEA test is recommended at baseline and every 3 to 6 months for 2 years [74], then every 6 months for a total of 5 years for patients with stage III disease and those with stage II disease if the clinician determines that the patient is a potential candidate for aggressive curative surgery [66, 74].

Colonoscopy is recommended at approximately 1 year after resection (or at 3-6 months post-resection if not performed pre-operatively because of an obstructing lesion). Repeat colonoscopy is typically recommended at 3 years, and then every 5 years thereafter, unless follow-up colonoscopy indicates advanced adenoma (villous polyp, polyp >1 cm, or higher-grade dysplasia), in which case colonoscopy should be repeated in 1 year [73]. More frequent colonoscopies may be indicated in patients who present with CRC before 50 years of age. Chest, abdominal, and pelvic CT scan are recommended annually for up to 5 years in patients with stage III disease and those with stage II disease at a high risk for recurrence [66, 75]. Routine CEA monitoring and CT scanning are not recommended beyond 5 years, routine use of PET/CT to monitor for disease recurrence is not recommended [75]. The CT that accompanies a PET/CT is usually a noncontrast CT, and therefore not of ideal quality for routine surveillance.

Panel recommendations for surveillance of patients with stage IV CRC with NED after curative-intent surgery and subsequent adjuvant treatment are similar to those listed for patients with stage II/III disease, except that certain evaluations are performed more frequently.

References

[1] Jemal A, Bray F, Center MM, Ferlay J, Ward E, Forman D. Global cancer statistics. CA *Cancer J. Clin.* 2011; 61: 69-90.

[2] Dušek J, Mužík D. Epidemiology of colorectal cancer: international comparisonL. Malúšková Institute of Biostatistics and Analyses, Masaryk University, Brno, Czech Republic.

[3] Ferlay J, Shin HR, Bray F, Forman D, Mathers C, Parkin DM. GLOBOCAN 2008 v1.2, Cancer Incidence and Mortality Worldwide: IARC CancerBase No. 10 [online]. *International Agency for Research on Cancer,* Lyon (France) 2010. Available from www: http://globocan.iarc.fr.

[4] Ferlay J, Parkin DM, Curado MP, Bray F, Edwards B, Shin HR, Forman D. *Cancer Incidence in Five Continents*, Volumes I to IX: IARC CancerBase No. 9 [online]. *International Agency for Research on Cancer,* Lyon (France) 2010. Available from www:http://ci5.iarc.fr.

[5] Ferlay J, Autier P, Boniol M, Heanue M, Colombet M, Boyle P. Estimates of the cancer incidence and mortality in Europe in 2006, *Ann Oncol.* 2007; 18: 581–592.

[6] Köhne CH, Kretzschmar A, Wils J. First-line chemotherapy for colorectal carcinoma—we are making progress. *Onkologie.* 1998; 21: 280–289.

[7] Steinberg SM, Barkin JS, Kaplan RS, Stablein DM. Prognostic indicators of colon tumors. The Gastrointestinal Tumor Study Group experience. *Cancer.* 1986; 57: 1866–1870.

[8] Kemeny N, Braun DW Jr. Prognostic factors in advanced colorectal carcinoma. Importance of lactic dehydrogenase level, performance status, and white blood cell count. *Am. J. Med* 1983; 74: 786–794.

[9] Graf W, Bergstrom R, Pahlman L, Glimelius B. Appraisal of a model for prediction of prognosis in advanced colorectal cancer. *Eur. J. Cancer* 1994; 30A: 453–457.

[10] Graf W, Glimelius B, Pahlman L, Bergstrom R. Determinants of prognosis in advanced colorectal cancer. *Eur. J. Cancer* 1991; 27: 1119–1123.

[11] Díaz R, Aparicio J, Gironés R, Molina J, Palomar L, Segura A, Montalar J. Analysis of prognostic factors and applicability of Kohne's prognostic groups in patients with metastatic colorectal cancer treated with first-line irinotecan or oxaliplatin-based chemotherapy. *Clin. Colorectal Cancer.* 2005; 5: 197-202.

[12] Sanoff HK, Sargent D J, Campbell ME, Morton RF, Fuchs CS, Ramanathan RK, Williamson SK, Findlay BP, Pitot HC, Goldberg RM: Five-year data and prognostic factor analysis of oxaliplatin and irinotecan combination for advanced colorectal cancer: N9741. *J. Clin Oncol.* 2008; 26: 5721-5727.

[13] Chibaudel B, Tournigand C, Artru P, Andrè T, Cervantes A, Figer A, Lledo G, Flesch M, Buyse M, Mineur L, Carola E, Rivera F, Perez-Staub N, Louvet C, de Gramont A. Folfox in patients with metastatic colorectal cancer and high alkaline phosphatase level: an exploratory cohort of the GERCOR OPTIMOX 1 study. *Ann. Oncol* 2009; 20: 1383-1386.

[14] Desot E, de Mestier L, Volet J, Delmas C, Garcia B, Geoffroy P, Abdelli N, Baule M, Dubroeucq O, Marquis E, Bouché O. Prognostic factors in patients with non resectable metastatic colorectal cancer in the era of targeted biotherapies: relevance of Köhne's risk classification. *Dig Liver Dis.* 2013; 45: 330-335.

[15] Berretta M, Zanet E, Basile F, Ridolfo AL, Di Benedetto F, Bearz A, Berretta S, Nasti G, Tirelli U. HIV-positive patients with liver metastases from colorectal cancer deserve the same therapeutic approach as the general population. *Onkologie.* 2010; 33: 203-204.

[16] Berretta M, Lleshi A, Cappellani A, Bearz A, Spina M, Talamini R, Cacopardo B, Nunnari G, Montesarchio V, Izzi I, Lanzafame M, Nasti G, Basile F, Berretta S, Fisichella R, Schiantarelli C C, Garlassi E, Ridolfo A, Guella L, Tirelli U. Oxaliplatin based chemotherapy and concomitant highly active antiretroviral therapy in the treatment of 24 patients with colorectal cancer and HIV infection. *Curr. HIV Res.* 2010; 8: 218-222.

[17] Berretta M, Cappellani A, Di Benedetto F, Lleshi A, Talamini R, Canzonieri V, Zanet E, Bearz A, Nasti G, Lacchin T, Berretta S, Fisichella R, Balestreri L, Torresin A, Izzi I, Ortolani P, Tirelli U. Clinical presentation and outcome of colorectal cancer in HIV-positive patients: a clinical case-control study. *Onkologie*. 2009; 32: 319-324.

[18] Berretta M, Di Benedetto F, Bearz A, Simonelli C, Martellotta F, Del Ben C, Berretta S, Spina M, Tirelli U. FOLFOX-4 regimen with concomitant highly active antiretroviral therapy in metastatic colorectal cancer HIV-infected patients: a report of five cases and review of the literature. *Cancer Invest*. 2008; 26: 610-614.

[19] Di Benedetto F, D'Amico G, Spaggiari M, Tirelli U, Berretta M. Onco-surgical management of colo-rectal liver metastases in older patients: a new frontier in the 3rd millennium. *Anticancer Agents Med Chem*. 2013; 13: 1354-1363.

[20] Berretta M, Aprile G, Nasti G, Urbani M, Bearz A, Lutrino S, Foltran L, Ferrari L, Talamini R, Fiorica F, Lleshi A, Canzonieri V, Lestuzzi C, Borsatti E, Fisichella R, Tirelli U. Oxaliplapin and capecitabine (XELOX) based chemotherapy in the treatment of metastatic colorectal cancer: the right choice in elderly patients. *Anticancer Agents Med Chem*. 2013; 13:1344-1353.

[21] Berretta M, Di Benedetto F, Di Francia R, Lo Menzo E, Palmeri S, De Paoli P, Tirelli U. Colorectal cancer in elderly patients: from best supportive care to cure. *Anticancer Agents Med Chem*. 2013; 13: 1332-1343.

[22] Di Benedetto F, Berretta M, D'Amico G, Montalti R, De Ruvo N, Cautero N, Guerrini GP, Ballarin R, Spaggiari M, Tarantino G, Di Sandro S, Pecchi A, Luppi G, Gerunda GE. Liver resection for colorectal metastases in older adults: a paired matched analysis. *J. Am. Geriatr Soc*. 2011; 59: 2282-2290.

[23] Berretta M, Zanet E, Nasti G, Lleshi A, Frustaci S, Fiorica F, Bearz A, Talamini R, Lestuzzi C, Lazzarini R, Fisichella R, Cannizzaro R, Iaffaioli RV, Berretta S, Tirelli U. Oxaliplatin-based chemotherapy in the treatment of elderly patients with metastatic colorectal cancer (CRC). *Arch Gerontol Geriatr*. 2012; 55: 271-275.

[24] Berretta M, Cappellani A, Fiorica F, Nasti G, Frustaci S, Fisichella R, Bearz A, Talamini R, Lleshi A, Tambaro R, Cocciolo A, Ristagno M, Bolognese A, Basile F, Meneguzzo N, Berretta S, Tirelli U. FOLFOX4 in the treatment of metastatic colorectal cancer in elderly patients: a prospective study. *Arch Gerontol Geriatr*. 2011; 52: 89-93.

[25] Yonemura Y, Canbay E, Ishibashi H. Prognostic factors of peritoneal metastases from colorectal cancer following cytoreductive surgery and perioperative chemotherapy. *ScientificWorldJournal.* 2013; 2013: 978394.

[26] Marzouk O, Schofield J. Review of histopathological and molecular prognostic features in colorectal cancer. *Cancers* (Basel). 2011; 3: 2767-2810.

[27] Lastoria S, Piccirillo MC, Caracò C, Nasti G, Aloj L, Arrichiello C, de Lutio di Castelguidone E, Tatangelo F, Ottaiano A, Iaffaioli RV, Izzo F, Romano G, Giordano P, Signoriello S, Gallo C, Perrone F. Early PET/CT scan is more effective than response evaluation criteria in solid tumors in predicting outcome of patients with liver metastases from colorectal cancer treated with preoperative chemotherapy plus bevacizumab. *J. Nucl Med.* 2013; 54: 2062-2069.

[28] Celik B, Yalcin AD, Bisgin A, Dimitrakopoulou-Strauss A, Kargi A, Strauss LG. Level of TNF-related apoptosis-inducing-ligand and CXCL8 correlated with 2-[18F]Fluoro-2-deoxy-D-glucose uptake in anti-VEGF treated colon cancers. *Med. Sci Monit.* 2013; 19: 875-882.

[29] Selcukbiricik F, Bilici A, Tural D, Erdamar S, Soyluk O, Buyukunal E, Demirelli F, Serdengecti S. Are high initial CEA and CA 19-9 levels associated with the presence of K-ras mutation in patients with metastatic colorectal cancer? *Tumour Biol.* 2013; 34: 2233-2239.

[30] Baek JY, Yeo HY, Chang HJ, Kim KH, Kim SY, Park JW, Park SC, Choi HS, Kim DY, Oh JH. Serpin B5 is a CEA-interacting biomarker for colorectal cancer. *Int. J. Cancer.* 2014; 134: 1595-1604.

[31] Wang WS, Lin JK, Chiou TJ, Liu JH, Fan FS, Yen CC, Lin TC, Jiang JK, Yang SH, Wang HS, Chen PM. CA19-9 as the most significant prognostic indicator of metastatic colorectal cancer. *Hepatogastroenterology.* 2002; 49: 160-164.

[32] Mekenkamp LJ, Heesterbeek KJ, Koopman M, Tol J, Teerenstra S, Venderbosch S, Punt CJ, Nagtegaal ID. Mucinous adenocarcinomas: Poor prognosis in metastatic colorectal cancer. *Eur. J. Cancer.* 2012; 48: 501-509.

[33] Yamaguchi T, Taniguchi H, Fujita S, Sekine S, Yamamoto S, Akasu T, Kushima R, Tani T, Moriya Y, Shimoda T. Clinicopathological characteristics and prognostic factors of advanced colorectal mucinous adenocarcinoma. *Histopathology* 2012; 61: 162-169.

[34] Ilyas M, Straub J, Tomlinson IP, Bodmer WF. Genetic pathways in colorectal and other cancers. *Eur. J. Cancer.* 1999; 35: 335-351.

[35] Arteaga CL. Targeting HER1/EGFR: a molecular approach to cancer therapy. *Semin Oncol.* 2003; 30 (3 Suppl 7): 3-14.

[36] Arteaga CL. Overview of epidermal growth factor receptor biology and its role as a therapeutic target in human neoplasia. *Semin Oncol.* 2002; 29 (5 Suppl 14): 3-9.

[37] Volgelstein B, Kinzler KW. *The genetic basis of human cancer.* London (U.K.): McGraw-Hill, 1999: 565-587.

[38] Wan PT, Garnett MJ, Roe SM, Lee S, Niculescu-Duvaz D, Good VM, Jones CM, Marshall CJ, Springer CJ, Barford D, Marais R; Cancer Genome Project. Mechanism of activation of the RAF-ERK signaling pathway by oncogenic mutations of B-RAF. *Cell.* 2004; 116, 855-867.

[39] Benvenuti S, Sartore-Bianchi A, Di Nicolantonio F, Zanon C, Moroni M, Veronese S, Siena S, Bardelli A. Oncogenic activation of the RAS/RAF signaling pathway impairs the response of metastatic colorectal cancers to anti-epidermal growth factor receptor antibody therapies. *Cancer Res.* 2007; 67: 2643-2648.

[40] Souglakos J, Philips J, Wang R, Marwah S, Silver M, Tzardi M, Silver J, Ogino S, Hooshmand S, Kwak E, Freed E, Meyerhardt JA, Saridaki Z, Georgoulias V, Finkelstein D, Fuchs CS, Kulke MH, Shivdasani RA. Prognostic and predictive value of common mutations for treatment response and survival in patients with metastatic colorectal cancer. *Br. J. Cancer.* 2009; 101, 465-472.

[41] Karapetis CS, Khambata-Ford S, Jonker DJ, O'Callaghan CJ, Tu D, Tebbutt NC, Simes RJ, Chalchal H, Shapiro JD, Robitaille S, Price TJ, Shepherd L, Au HJ, Langer C, Moore MJ, Zalcberg JR. K-ras mutations and benefit from cetuximab in advanced colorectal cancer. *N. Engl J. Med.* 2008; 59: 1757-1765.

[42] Van Cutsem E, Köhne CH, Hitre E, Zaluski J, Chang Chien CR, Makhson A, D'Haens G, Pintér T, Lim R, Bodoky G, Roh JK, Folprecht G, Ruff P, Stroh C, Tejpar S, Schlichting M, Nippgen J, Rougier P. Cetuximab and chemotherapy as initial treatment for metastatic colorectal cancer. *N Engl. J. Med.* 2009; 360: 1408-1417.

[43] Bokemeyer C, Bondarenko I, Makhson A, Hartmann JT, Aparicio J, de Braud F, Donea S, Ludwig H, Schuch G, Stroh C, Loos AH, Zubel A, Koralewski P. Fluorouracil, leucovorin, and oxaliplatin with and without cetuximab in the firstline treatment of metastatic colorectal cancer. *J. Clin. Oncol.* 2009; 27: 663-671.

[44] Tol J, Nagtegaal ID, Punt CJ. BRAF mutation in metastatic colorectal cancer. *N Engl. J. Med.* 2009; 361: 98-99.

[45] Clarke PA. Kirsten ras mutations in patients with colorectal cancer: the multicenter ''RASCAL'' study. *J. Natl. Cancer Inst*. 1998; 90: 675-684.

[46] Yokota T. Are KRAS/BRAF mutations potent prognostic and/or predictive biomarkers in colorectal cancers? *Anticancer Agents Med Chem.* 2012; 12: 163-1.

[47] French AJ, Sargent DJ, Burgart LJ, Foster NR, Kabat BF, Goldberg R, Shepherd L, Windschitl HE, Thibodeau SN. Prognostic significance of defective mismatch repair and BRAF V600E in patients with colon cancer. *Clin. Cancer Res*. 2008; 14: 3408-3415.

[48] Kakar S, Deng G, Sahai V, Matsuzaki K, Tanaka H, Miura S, Kim YS. Clinicopathologic characteristics, CpG island methylator phenotype, and BRAF mutations in microsatellite-stable colorectal cancers without chromosomal instability. *Arch Pathol Lab Med*. 2008; 132: 958-964.

[49] Ogino S, Nosho K, Kirkner GJ, Kawasaki T, Meyerhardt JA, Loda M, Giovannucci EL, Fuchs CS. CpG island methylator phenotype, microsatellite instability, BRAF mutation and clinical outcome in colon cancer. *Gut* 2009; 58: 90-96.

[50] Roth AD, Tejpar S, Delorenzi M, Yan P, Fiocca R, Klingbiel D, Dietrich D, Biesmans B, Bodoky G, Barone C, Aranda E, Nordlinger B, Cisar L, Labianca R, Cunningham D, Van Cutsem E, Bosman F. Prognostic role of KRAS and BRAF in stage II and III resected colon cancer: results of the translational study on the PETACC-3, EORTC 40993, SAKK 60-00 trial. *J. Clin. Oncol*. 2010; 28: 466-474.

[51] Irahara N, Baba Y, Nosho K, Shima K, Yan L, Dias-Santagata D, Iafrate AJ, Fuchs CS, Haigis KM, Ogino S. NRAS Mutations Are Rare in Colorectal Cancer. *Diagn Mol Pathol*. 2010; 19: 157–163.

[52] Tejpar S, Celik I, Schlichting M, Sartorius U, Bokemeyer C, Van Cutsem E. Association of KRAS G13D tumor mutations with outcome in patients with metastatic colorectal cancer treated with first-line chemotherapy with or without cetuximab. *J. Clin. Oncol*. 2012; 30: 3570-3577.

[53] Souglakos J, Philips J, Wang R, Marwah S, Silver M, Tzardi M, Silver J, Ogino S, Hooshmand S, Kwak E, Freed E, Meyerhardt JA, Saridaki Z, Georgoulias V, Finkelstein D, Fuchs CS, Kulke MH, Shivdasani RA. Prognostic and predictive value of common mutations for treatment response and survival in patients with metastatic colorectal cancer. *Br. J. Cancer*. 2009 Aug 4;101(3):465-72.

[54] Di Nicolantonio F, Martini M, Molinari F, Sartore-Bianchi A, Arena S, Saletti P, De Dosso S, Mazzucchelli L, Frattini M, Siena S, Bardelli A.

Wild-type BRAF is required for response to panitumumab or cetuximab in metastatic colorectal cancer. *J. Clin. Oncol.* 2008; 26: 5705-5712.

[55] Karapetis CS, Khambata-Ford S, Jonker DJ, O'Callaghan CJ, Tu D, Tebbutt NC, Simes RJ, Chalchal H, Shapiro JD, Robitaille S, Price TJ, Shepherd L, Au HJ, Langer C, Moore MJ, Zalcberg JR. K-ras mutations and benefit from cetuximab in advanced colorectal cancer. *N. Engl. J. Med.* 2008; 359: 1757-1765.

[56] Douillard JY, Oliner KS, Siena S, Tabernero J, Burkes R, Barugel M, Humblet Y, Bodoky G, Cunningham D, Jassem J, Rivera F, Kocákova I, Ruff P, Błasińska-Morawiec M, Šmakal M, Canon JL, Rother M, Williams R, Rong A, Wiezorek J, Sidhu R, Patterson SD. Panitumumab-FOLFOX4 treatment and RAS mutations in colorectal cancer. *N. Engl. J. Med.* 2013; 369: 1023-1034.

[57] Atreya CE, Sangale Z, Xu N, Matli MR, Tikishvili E, Welbourn W, Stone S, Shokat KM, Warren RS. PTEN expression is consistent in colorectal cancer primaries and metastases and associates with patient survival. *Cancer Med.* 2013; 2: 496-506.

[58] Lim SW, Kim HR, Kim HY, Huh JW, Kim YJ, Shin JH, Suh SP, Ryang DW, Kim HR, Shin MG. Over-expression of Her-2 in colorectal cancer tissue, but not in serum, constitutes an independent worse prognostic factor. *Cell Oncol* (Dordr). 2013; 36: 311-321.

[59] Karagkounis G, Torbenson MS, Daniel HD, Azad NS, Diaz LA Jr, Donehower RC, Hirose K, Ahuja N, Pawlik TM, Choti MA. Incidence and prognostic impact of KRAS and BRAF mutation in patients undergoing liver surgery for colorectal metastases. *Cancer.* 2013; 119: 4137-4144.

[60] NCCN Guidelines Version 3.2014, Colon Cancer.

[61] Sargent D, Sobrero A, Grothey A, O'Connell MJ, Buyse M, Andre T, Zheng Y, Green E, Labianca R, O'Callaghan C, Seitz JF, Francini G, Haller D, Yothers G, Goldberg R, de Gramont A. Evidence for cure by adjuvant therapy in colon cancer: observations based on individual patient data from 20,898 patients on 18 randomized trials. *J. Clin. Oncol.* 2009; 27: 872-877.

[62] Seo SI, Lim SB, Yoon YS, Kim CW, Yu CS, Kim TW, Kim JH, Kim JC. Comparison of recurrence patterns between ≤5 years and >5 years after curative operations in colorectal cancer patients. *J. Surg. Oncol.* 2013; 108: 9-13.

[63] Pietra N, Sarli L, Costi R, Ouchemi C, Grattarola M, Peracchia A. Role of follow-up in management of local recurrences of colorectal cancer: a

prospective, randomized study. *Dis. Colon Rectum.* 1998; 41: 1127-1133.

[64] Rodríguez-Moranta F, Saló J, Arcusa A, Boadas J, Piñol V, Bessa X, Batiste-Alentorn E, Lacy AM, Delgado S, Maurel J, Piqué JM, Castells A. Postoperative surveillance in patients with colorectal cancer who have undergone curative resection: a prospective, multicenter, randomized, controlled trial. *J. Clin. Oncol.* 2006; 24: 386-393.

[65] Secco GB, Fardelli R, Gianquinto D, Bonfante P, Baldi E, Ravera G, Derchi L, Ferraris R. Efficacy and cost of risk-adapted follow-up in patients after colorectal cancer surgery: a prospective, randomized and controlled trial. *Eur. J. Surg Oncol.* 2002; 28: 418-423.

[66] Desch CE, Benson AB 3rd, Somerfield MR, Flynn PJ, Krause C, Loprinzi CL, Minsky BD, Pfister DG, Virgo KS, Petrelli NJ; American Society of Clinical Oncology. Colorectal cancer surveillance: 2005 update of an American Society of Clinical Oncology practice guideline. J Clin Oncol. 2005; 23: 8512-8519. *Erratum in: J. Clin Oncol.* 2006 Mar 1;24(7):1224.

[67] Figueredo A, Rumble RB, Maroun J, Earle CC, Cummings B, McLeod R, Zuraw L, Zwaal C; Gastrointestinal Cancer Disease Site Group of Cancer Care Ontario's Program in Evidence-based Care. Follow-up of patients with curatively resected colorectal cancer: a practice guideline. *BMC Cancer.* 2003; 3: 26.

[68] Jeffery M, Hickey BE, Hider PN. Follow-up strategies for patients treated for non-metastatic colorectal cancer. *Cochrane Database Syst Rev.* 2007; (1): CD002200.

[69] Renehan AG, Egger M, Saunders MP, O'Dwyer ST. Impact on survival of intensive follow up after curative resection for colorectal cancer: systematic review and meta-analysis of randomised trials. *BMJ.* 2002; 324: 813.

[70] Tsikitis VL, Malireddy K, Green EA, Christensen B, Whelan R, Hyder J, Marcello P, Larach S, Lauter D, Sargent DJ, Nelson H. Postoperative surveillance recommendations for early stage colon cancer based on results from the clinical outcomes of surgical therapy trial. *J. Clin. Oncol.* 2009; 27: 3671-3676.

[71] Guyot F, Faivre J, Manfredi S, Meny B, Bonithon-Kopp C, Bouvier AM. Time trends in the treatment and survival of recurrences from colorectal cancer. *Ann. Oncol.* 2005; 16: 756-761.

[72] Primrose JN, Perera R, Gray A, Rose P, Fuller A, Corkhill A, George S, Mant D; FACS Trial Investigators. Effect of 3 to 5 years of scheduled

CEA and CT follow-up to detect recurrence of colorectal cancer: the FACS randomized clinical trial. *JAMA*. 2014; 311: 263-270.

[73] Rex DK, Kahi CJ, Levin B, Smith RA, Bond JH, Brooks D, Burt RW, Byers T, Fletcher RH, Hyman N, Johnson D, Kirk L, Lieberman DA, Levin TR, O'Brien MJ, Simmang C, Thorson AG, Winawer SJ; American Cancer Society; US Multi-Society Task Force on Colorectal Cancer. Guidelines for colonoscopy surveillance after cancer resection: a consensus update by the American Cancer Society and the US Multi-Society Task Force on Colorectal Cancer. *Gastroenterology*. 2006; 130: 1865-1871.

[74] Locker GY, Hamilton S, Harris J, Jessup JM, Kemeny N, Macdonald JS, Somerfield MR, Hayes DF, Bast RC Jr; ASCO. ASCO 2006 update of recommendations for the use of tumor markers in gastrointestinal cancer. *J. Clin. Oncol.* 2006; 24: 5313-5327.

[75] Pfister DG, Benson AB 3rd, Somerfield MR. Clinical practice. Surveillance strategies after curative treatment of colorectal cancer. *N. Engl. J. Med.* 2004; 350: 2375-2382.

In: Prognostic and Predictive Response ... ISBN: 978-1-63463-545-5
Editors: V. Canzonieri and M. Berretta

Chapter 3

Gastric Cancer: Prognostic and Predictive Response Therapy Factors

C. De Divitiis[1], *V. Canzonieri*[2], *R. Cannizzaro*[3], *G. Nasti*[4], *P. De Paoli*[5], *R. Fisichella*[6] *and M. Berretta*[7,8,*]

[1]Medical Oncology SUN of Naples and IRCCS Fondazione Pascale Napoli, Italy
[2]Gastroenterology Division, CRO – National Cancer Institute, IRCCS Aviano, Italy
[3]Division of Pathology, CRO - National Cancer Institute, IRCCS Aviano, Italy
[4]Medical Oncology IRCCS Fondazione Pascale Napoli, Italy
[5]Scientific Directorate, CRO - National Cancer Institute, IRCCS Aviano, Italy
[6]Department of Surgery, University of Catania, Catania Italy
[7]Department of Medical Oncology, CRO – National Cancer Institute, IRCCS Aviano, Italy
[8]Euro-Mediterranean Institute of Science and Technology (IEMEST), Palermo, Italy

[*] Corresponding author: Massimiliano Berretta, MD, Ph.D. Department of Medical Oncology, National Cancer Institute - I.R.C.C.S. Via F. Gallini 2 Aviano (PN), 33081 Italy. Phone +39 434 659724, mobile +39 333 3914670, fax +39 0434 659531.

Abstract

Despite the recent progress in the development of new therapeutic strategies and in early diagnosis, the prognosis of gastric cancer continues to be poor, with < 20% of patients surviving at 5 years.

With these perspectives, it becomes of big importance to identify factors helping to predict survival and/or response to treatment, to choose better among the available therapeutic tools.

Introduction

Gastric cancer is one of the most common cancers worldwide. Approximately 21,600 patients are diagnosed annually in the United States, of whom 10,990 are expected to die [1–6].

Gastric cancer used to be the leading cause of cancer deaths in the world until the 1980s when it was overtaken by lung cancer. The worldwide incidence of gastric cancer has declined rapidly over the recent few decades. Part of the decline may be due to the recognition of certain risk factors such as H. pylori and other dietary and environmental risks [7–10]. However, the decline clearly began before the discovery of H. pylori. The decline first took place in countries with low gastric cancer incidence such as the United States (beginning in the 1930s), while the decline in countries with high incidence like Japan was slower [11]. In the United Kingdom, there was a consistent decline in incidence of gastric cancer, with a reduction in RR from 1.14 in 1971 to 1975 to 0.84 in 1996 to 2000 in men, and 1.18 in 1971 to 1975 to 0.81 in 1996 to 2000 in women [12, 13]. In China, the decline was less dramatic than other countries; despite an overall decrease in gastric cancer incidence, an increase has been observed in the oldest and the youngest group, and a less remarkable decline has been observed among women than in men. Of note is that the age of onset of developing gastric cancer in Chinese population is younger than that in the West [14]. In the United States, risk factors for noncardia gastric cancer include male gender, non-white race, and older age. Between 1977 and 2006, the incidence rate for non-cardia gastric cancer in the United States declined among all race and age groups except for whites aged 29 to 39 years for whom it increased [15-17]. The rise in incidence of non - cardia gastric cancer among those at 25 to 39 years is noteworthy since this may signal the introduction of new environmental factors.

An interesting hypothesis is that the popularization of refrigerators marks a pivotal point for the decline. Refrigerators improved the storage of food, thereby reducing salt-based preservation of food and preventing bacterial and fungal contamination. Refrigeration also allowed for fresh food and vegetables to be more readily available, which may be a valuable source of antioxidants important for cancer prevention [18, 19].

Clinical Prognostic Factors

Despite the recent progress in the development of new therapeutic strategies and in early diagnosis, the prognosis of gastric cancer continues to be poor, with < 20% of patients surviving at 5 years [20-22].

Within this framework, identifying factors helping to predict survival and response to treatment is a crucial issue and may suggest an appropriate strategy among the available therapeutic options. The TNM stage is one of the most important prognostic tool for gastric cancer.

The prognosis of patients with gastric cancer is related to tumor extent and includes both nodal involvement and direct tumor extension beyond the gastric wall. Tumor grade may also provide some prognostic information [23, 24].

In localized distal gastric cancer, more than 50% of patients can be cured. However, early-stage disease accounts for only 10% to 20% of all cases diagnosed in the United States. The remaining patients present with metastatic disease in either regional or distant sites. The overall survival rate in these patients at 5 years ranges from almost no survival for patients with disseminated disease to almost 50% survival for patients with localized distal gastric cancers confined to resectable regional disease. Even with apparent localized disease, the 5-year survival rate of patients with proximal gastric cancer is only 10% to 15%. Although the treatment of patients with disseminated gastric cancer may result in palliation of symptoms and some prolongation of survival, long remissions are uncommon.

Recurrence following surgery is a major problem, and is often the ultimate cause of death. Residual tumor after gastric resection with curative intent is categorized by a system known as R classification and indicates the amount of residual disease left after tumor resection: R0 indicates no gross or microscopic residual tumor, R1 indicates microscopic residual tumor, and R2 shows macroscopic residual disease. This obvious and important prognostic factor was not always reported in the past, making interpretation of survival results difficult [25].

Two prognostic factors are standard on a type C basis: the degree of penetration of the tumor through the gastric wall, and the presence of lymph node involvement. These two factors also form the basis for all staging systems developed for this disease. The relationship between T stage and survival is well defined. Several reports from Japan, Europe, and the United States have demonstrated the significant prognostic importance of advanced T stage [26]. In the past, the N stage classification was based on the anatomical location of lymph nodes. Although the prognostic significance of such a classification may be relevant, it is very complicated for practice. In 1997, the AJCC/UICC N stage was changed and became based on the number of positive lymph nodes [27]. This new classification has fewer methodological problems, and it seems more reproducible provided that a minimum of 15 nodes are removed and analyzed.

Apart from TNM classification and R0 resection, many other factors have been considered for prognostic purposes.

Most multivariate analyses have shown no effect on prognosis of the tumor histological classification proposed by the WHO, independent of stage, with the exception of the rare small cell carcinoma of the stomach, which has an unfavourable prognosis [28]. Other histological prognostic factors were considered the Laurén classification (intestinal or diffuse type), or the Ming classification (expanding or infiltrating type). For all stage groupings, grading correlates with outcome [29, 30]. The Lauren's classification differentiates gastric cancers into two major types: intestinal or diffuse.

This classification, based on tumor histology, characterizes two varieties of gastric adenocarcinomas, which have different pathology, epidemiology, aetiologies, and behaviour. The intestinal type consists of a differentiated cancer with a tendency to form glands.

By contrast, the diffuse form exhibits low cell cohesion and tends to replace the gastric mucosa by signet-ring cells. About 16% of cases will be unclassifiable or of mixed type. Ming proposed a classification favourable expanding type, and the poor prognosis infiltrating type [31, 32].

Macroscopic tumor configuration types as described by Borrmann has been shown to have prognostic significance in several large studies; I and II Borrmann types (polypoid and ulcerating cancers) seem to have a better prognosis than III and IV Borrmann types (infiltrating cancers). However, the prognostic value of tumor configuration has not been confirmed in other studies. Studies in Asia have questioned the dictum that signet ring cell carcinoma (SRC) has a worse prognosis than other forms of gastric cancer [33].

In a study, Sharven Taghavi et al. determined differences in presentation and outcomes between SRC and gastric adenocarcinoma (AC) in the United States. They reviewed 10,246 cases of patients with gastric cancer, including 2,666 of SRC and 7,580 of AC.

SRC presented in younger patients and less often in men. SRC patients were more frequently black, Asian, American Indian/Alaska Native, or Hispanic. SRC was more likely to be stage T3-4 (45.8% *v* 33.3%), have lymph node spread (59.7% *v* 51.8%), and distant metastases (40.2% *v* 37.6%). SRC was more likely to be found in the lower (30.7% *v* 24.2%) and middle stomach (30.6% *v* 20.7%). Median survival was not different between the two (AC, 14.0 months *v* SRC, 13.0 months; *P*_.073). Multivariable analyses demonstrated SRC was not associated with mortality (hazard ratio [HR], 1.05; 95% CI, 0.96 to 1.11; *P* _ .150). Mortality was associated with age (HR, 1.01; 95% CI, 1.01 to 1.02; *P* _ .001), black race (HR, 1.10; 95% CI, 1.01 to 1.20; *P* _ .026), and tumor grade. Variables associated with lower mortality risk included Asian race (HR, 0.83; 95% CI, 0.77 to 0.91; *P*_.001) and surgery (HR, 0.37; 95% CI, 0.34 to 0.39; *P* _ .001). In the United States, SRC significantly differs from AC in extent of disease at presentation. However, when adjusted for stage, SRC does not portend a worse prognosis.

The adverse prognostic factor of tumor size is controversial. Tumor site has been shown to be an independent prognostic factor in gastric carcinoma, with proximal carcinomas (i.e., tumors of the upper third of the stomach, including the gastric cardia and gastroesophageal junction) having a poorer prognosis than distal cancers [33].

Lymphatic, venous, or perineural invasion have been shown to be adverse prognostic factors [34]. Several studies have reported a positive surgical resection margin associated with a significant decrease in overall survival [35–38]. The ratio of lymph nodes metastases (number of metastatic lymph nodes to the total number of dissected lymph nodes) appears to be an important prognostic factor and the best classification factor for lymph node metastasis [39]. Different survival rates have been reported between patients having undergone surgical intervention for the treatment of gastric carcinoma in Japan and Western countries. However, when using a similar staging classification and similar prognostic characteristics, the prognosis for gastric cancer in Japan and Germany may be the same [40]. Tumor volume, measured from serial tissue sections of gastric carcinoma by using a computer graphics analysis, seems to be of prognostic significance. In a recent report by Maehara et al. [41], multivariate analysis revealed that the 10 factors of depth of invasion, lymph node metastasis, lymph node dissection, tumor size, liver metastasis, peritoneal dissemination, lymphatic invasion, vascular invasion, lesion in the whole stomach, and lesion in the middle stomach were independent factors for determining the prognosis.

Although most reports [42] have suggested a dismal prognosis for young patients with gastric cancer, one study has suggested that young patients (< or =39 years) do not have a worse prognosis than older patients. Women appeared to have a better prognosis than men in one study [43], but this was not confirmed in other reports [44].

According to somc studics [45], oldcr paticnts havc bccn rcportcd to havc a poorer prognosis than younger patients, because they have more advanced disease stage at the time of diagnosis and a lower rate of curative resection. Also, other causes such cardiovascular disease, diabetics, other gerontological medical problems, alterations in the immune system, malnutrition have been suggested to reflect the increased operative mortality and shortened long term survival in older patients.

Prognostic Serum Markers

Due to their low sensitivity and specificity in detecting early primary tumors, classic biomarkers have shown little benefit as a method for screening in the general population. However, these markers may be used clinically for the monitoring of tumor recurrence or may be used as prognostic factors because it higher levels has been normally observed in advanced disease. The introduction of new techniques as polymerase chain reaction (PCR) may increase the sensibility of detection of these markers respect common immunoassays.

Carcinoembryonic Antigen (CEA)

Preoperative serum CEA levels have a predictive value in determining tumor stage and prognostic information for patients with potentially resectable gastric cancer during the preoperative period [46]. Curatively resected gastric cancer patients with higher preoperative plasma CEA levels have a poorer prognosis than those with lower levels, despite the adjustment for the effects of major prognostic factors [47–49]. Others authors have found that higher CEA levels in peritoneal washings in gastric cancer patients at the time of laparotomy are prognostic of poor survival [50, 51].

Chung et al. [52] reported higher CEA serum levels in advanced gastric cancer of intestinal-type. Kodama et al. [53] confirmed a low positive rate of CEA serum levels in early gastric cancers, similarly to Ca19.9 and Ca72.4. Ucar et al. [54] demonstrated a correlation between CEA positivity and the presence of liver metastases.

Nakanishi et al. [55] demonstrated a higher frequency of peritoneal metastases in patients with positive real time-PCR analysis for CEA transcripts in peritoneal washes of gastric cancer patients.

Carbohydrate Antigen (CA) 19-9

Kodama et al. [53] studies showed a low positive rate for Ca19.9 in early gastric cancer. Ucar et al. [54] reported a more frequent significant Ca19.9 serum positivity in patients with lymph nodes, peritoneal and serosal involvement.

Carbohydrate Antigen (Ca) 72-4

The 72.4 carbohydrate epitope, contained in highmolecular weight mucin-type glycoprotein, called TAG-72, is detected by monoclonal antibodies CC49 and B72-3. Kodama et al. [53] demonstrated a higher positive rate of serum expression for Ca 72.4 respect CEA and Ca19.9 in advanced gastric cancer, but not in early gastric cancer.

Moreover, a higher positive rate of expression was seen in the presence of peritoneal dissemination and a first elevation prior to other markers in the presence of recurrence.

Mattar et al. [56] confirmed the increased serum positive expression of Ca 72.4 in advanced gastric disease. Ucar et al. [54] showed a more frequent significant Ca 72.4 positivity in patients with lymph nodes, peritoneal and liver involvement, and described Ca 72.4 as the only independent prognostic factor for survival among other markers such as CEA, Ca19.9, αFP.

Fernandes et al. [57] showed a significant correlation between high levels of Ca 72.4 in peritoneal washing and lymph nodes metastasis and serosa involvement by gastric cancer and also with more advanced stage of gastric carcinoma. The levels of Ca 72.4 in the blood correlates significantly with only lymph nodes involvement by gastric carcinoma.

Prognostic Tissue Factors

In the last decades, many studies have suggested the role that genetic alterations may have in the development and progression of gastric cancer [58]. Molecular pathology may be helpful not only to understand the disease pathogenesis, but also to give useful prognostic molecular markers.

Biological prognostic factors are often derived from the genetic process, which is thought to represent a crucial step to gastric cancer (HER2, E-cadherin, EGFR, DNA copy number changes, microsatellite instability, and changes in expression of several factors including thymidilate synthase, beta-catenin, mucin antigen, p53, COX-2, matrix metalloproteinases, and vascular endothelial growth factor receptor). Some of these potential prognostic factors can also be predictive of response to therapy as they are a molecular target either to chemotherapeutics or to biologic/targeted therapies, such as trastuzumab in HER2-positive tumors.

Overexpression of p53 as demonstrated by immunohistochemistry has been reported in 17–91% of invasive tumors, whereas the reported incidence pf p53 mutations in invasive carcinomas ranges from 0 to 77% [59]. The assessment of the role of p53 in gastric cancer in relation to prognosis has produced conflicting result [60–64]. Published studies have reported conflicting and even contradictory results since they have involved immunohistochemical detection of the protein, which has been performed with different antibodies, detection techniques, or methods of interpretation. Other suggested biological prognostic factors were p21 expression, VEGF expression, overexpression of EGF-r, cyclin D2 overexpression, BAT-26 alterations, uPA (urokinase-type plasminogen activator) and PAI-1 (PA inhibitor), the serum level of soluble receptor for IL-2 (SolIL-2R), or some proliferation-related factors, such as Sphase fraction, Ki-67 or proliferating cell nuclear antigen (PCNA) [65]. Recent data on the correlation between molecular markers and response to chemotherapy are still controversial [66]. Using immunohistochemical p53 analysis of pre-treatment endoscopical samples, two studies have reported a relationship between p53 staining and response to chemotherapy. Thymidylate synthase expression seemed to be related to response to chemotherapy [69, 70].

A gene potentially involved in chemoresistance, ERCC-1 (excision repair cross-complementing), has been shown to be more highly expressed in non-responsive gastric cancer patients than in responsive patients.

Thus, these data arise from retrospective studies, and well designed, prospective trial are warranted to further define the role of molecular markers in predicting response and survival of patients with gastric cancer.

The cadherins are a major class of adhesion molecules that play an important role in the homotypic cell-cell adhesion and, hence, cancer cell metastasis and invasion. E-cadherin is a member of the cadherin family and is expressed on all epithelial cells. The invasiveness of epithelial tumor cell lines could be inhibited in vitro by transfection with E-cadherin cDNA, and the invasiveness of these cell lines were induced again by exposure to anti–E-cadherin monoclonal antibodies. Underexpression of the E-cadherin molecule has been found in various malignancies, and it has the potential value of being a prognostic factor. In addition to its role in metastasis, E-cadherin is one of the most important candidate genes in gastric carcinogenesis. Somatic mutations of the E-cadherin gene have been identified in more than 50% of diffuse types of gastric cancer. According to Knudson's two-hits theory, somatic mutation of E-cadherin is the first of the two hits mechanisms for the silencing of the molecule, whereas methylation of E-cadherin has recently been shown to act as the second hit. In fact, methylation of Ecadherin has recently been shown to be the second genetic hit 9 in gastric carcinogenesis.

Serum soluble E-cadherin is the degradation product of the cellular E-cadherin molecule. It is found in the circulation of normal individuals and is particularly elevated in patients with malignancies. Gofuku et al. 10 showed that the concentration was significantly elevated in 67% of patients with gastric cancer. Annie On – On Chan et al. found that high concentration of serum soluble E-cadherin was associated with inoperability/palliative treatment and lymph node metastasis [72-75]. Annie On – On Chan et al. have also studied the correlation between serum level of soluble E-cadherin and the protein expression by immunohistochemical staining:they found that soluble E-cadherin is a potentially valuable pre-therapeutic factor in predicting long-term survival in patients with gastric cancer. By using a pre-therapeutic level greater than 10,000, they were able to predict that 90% of patients would have a survival time < 3 years. Further prospective study is required to investigate the value of soluble E-cadherin to predict recurrence.

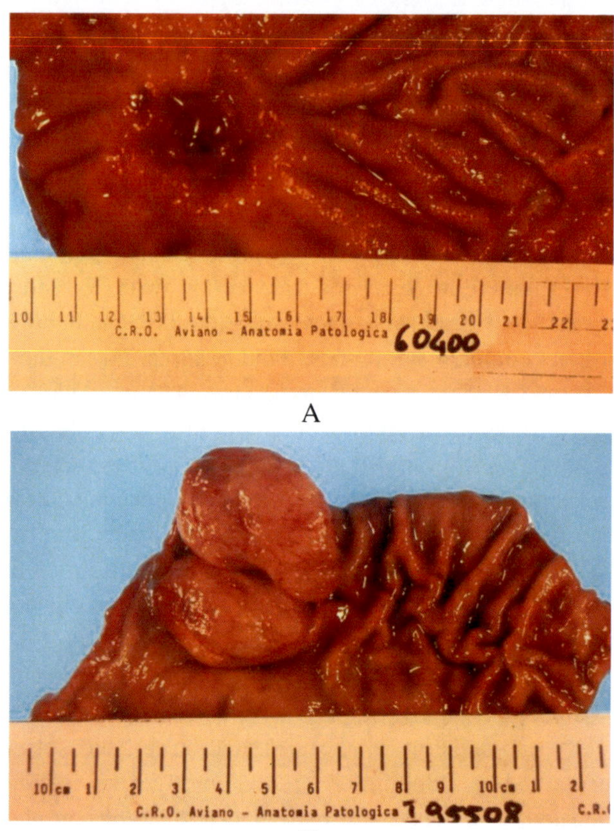

Figure 1. A. Gross appearances of a gastric ulcerated cancer. B. Gross appearance of a gastric polypoid cancer.

Predictive Tissue and Clinical Factors

In gastric carcinomas (GCs), HER1 and HER2 overexpression is thought to be a prognostic factor and a target of novel biologic agents.

The HER2 protein (p185, HER2/neu, ErbB-2) is an 185-kDa trans-membrane tyrosine kinase (TK) receptor and a member of the epidermal growth factor receptors (EGFRs) family.

This family is composed of four members: HER1 (also known as the EGFR), HER2, HER3 (also termed ErbB-3), and HER4 (also termed ErbB-4). These receptors share the same molecular structure with an extracellular ligand-binding domain, a short transmembrane domain, and an intracellular domain with TK activity (excepting the HER3). The binding of different ligands to the extracellular domain initiates a signal transduction cascade that can influence many aspects of tumor cell biology, including cell proliferation, apoptosis, adhesion, migration, and differentiation.

Ligand binding induces EGFR homodimerization as well as heterodimerization with other types of HER proteins. HER2 does not bind to any known ligand, but it is the preferred heterodimerization partner for other members of the HER family. HER2 is encoded by a gene located on chromosome 17q21. The HER2 gene, located adjacent to the topoisomerase IIa genes, is related to the oncogene v-erbB of the avian erythroblastosis virus.

In carcinomas, HER2 acts as an oncogene mainly because high level amplification of the gene induces protein overexpression in the cellular membrane and subsequent acquisition of advantageous properties for a malignant cell.

Recent studies indicate a role of HER2 in the development of numerous types of human cancer. HER2 overexpression and/or amplification have been detected in 10%-34% of invasive breast cancers and correlate with the clinical outcome, confer poor prognosis, and constitute also a predictive factor of poor response to chemotherapy and endocrine therapy.

HER2 overexpression and/or amplification have also been observed in colon, bladder, ovarian, endometrial, lung, uterine cervix, head and neck, esophageal, and gastric carcinomas.

Trastuzumab is a monoclonal antibody which specifically targets HER2 protein by directly binding the extracellular domain of the receptor. Trastuzumab enhances survival rates in both primary and metastatic HER2-positive breast cancer patients. The efficacy of trastuzumab in breast cancer patients has led to investigate its antitumor activity in patients with HER2-positive cancers, including gastric adenocarcinomas.

However, in gastric cancer, the clinical significance of such overexpression is not yet fully clear, and not all studies have shown an association between HER2 overexpression and poor prognosis.

Table 1. HER2 espression and clinicohistologic characteristics

Author	*n*	Histologic type				Localization			Method
		Intestinal (%)	Diffuse (%)	Mixed/unknown (%)	*P*	GEJ (%)	Gastric (%)	*P*	
Tanner et al. [39]	231	21.5	2	5	0.005	24	12	–	CISH
Gravalos et al. [28]	166	16	7	14	0.27	25	9.5	0.01	IHC, FISH
Lordick et al. [31]	1527	34	6	20	–	32	18	–	IHC, FISH

GEJ, gastroesophageal junction; CISH, chromogenic in situ hybridization; IHC, immunohistochemisry.

Although the effect of HER3 or HER4 expression in GC has not been clarified, HER3 expression is frequently observed in advanced gastric tumors with poor prognosis, and *HER4* gene expression seems to be higher in tumor tissue in comparison with adjacent gastric mucosa.

Some studies indicate that all members of the HER family are expressed in GC [76–85]. Furthermore, expression of HER2 and HER3 is a significant predictor of poor survival in GC and predictor of response to trastuzumab. Therefore, the development of HER-targeted agents and agents targeting downstream signaling pathways provides new possibilities in the treatment of GC.

There is increasing recognition of the existence of intratumoral heterogeneity of the human epidermal growth factor receptor (HER2), which affects interpretation of HER2 positivity in clinical practice and may have implications for patient prognosis and treatment.

The only targeted therapy approved in gastric cancer is trastuzumab. The Phase III ToGA trial [76-86] reported an increase in overall survival for patients with human EGF receptor (HER)2-positive gastric cancer treated with chemotherapy and trastuzumab compared to chemotherapy alone.

HER2, a component of the EGFR family associated with a poor prognosis in GC, predicts sensitivity to trastuzumab.

In the TOGA database, HER2 was positive in 22% of tumors (34% of intestinal type vs. 6% diffuse type and 20% mixed types). Furthermore, the highest rate was observed in 34% of GEJ tumors and 20% of GC samples. ToGA trial evaluated whether trastuzumab added to cisplatin and fluoropyrimidine could improve the efficacy of chemotherapy in HER2-positive advanced GC patients. The HER2 overexpression was defined as immunohistochemistry (IHC) 3+ and/or fluorescent in situ hybridization (FISH) positivity: therefore, the enrolment of patients was allowed with a FISH positivity with IHC 0 or 1+. The primary endpoint was OS. Secondary endpoints were PFS, time to progression (TTP), ORR, disease control, duration of response, and QoL. Of 3807 patients screened, 810 were HER2-positive (IHC 3+ and/or FISH+) and 584 were randomized between chemotherapy alone (290) or chemotherapy plus trastuzumab (294). Trastuzumab improved the median OS when compared with chemotherapy alone (13.8 vs 11.1 months; hazard ratio (HR) 0.74; $p < 0.0046$); PFS (HR 0.71; $p < 0.0002$), TTP (HR 0.70; $p < 0.0003$), ORR (OR 1.70; $p < 0.0017$) and QoL were also improved in the trastuzumab arm.

The best OS improvement was observed in IHC 2+/FISH+ or IHC 3+ patients: 16 months in the trastuzumab arm and 11.8 months in the chemotherapy alone arm (HR 0.65).

The toxicity was very mild, and no differences were recorded in the rate of cardiac adverse events between the two arms. Therefore, trastuzumab was approved in combination with cisplatin and fluoropyrimidines for metastatic untreated HER2-positive GC. HER2 status should be assessed routinely by primary IHC: tumors with IHC 3+ score are eligible for trastuzumab.

Samples with an equivocal IHC 2+ score should be retested using FISH: patients whose tumors score IHC2+/FISH+ are eligible for trastuzumab. According to these recommendations, ~16% of advanced GC patients are suitable for anti-HER2 therapy. Accurate HER2 testing in gastric cancer is therefore necessary.

The role of HER2 as a prognostic factor in gastric cancer has been controversial in the past because some of the initial studies failed to find an association with prognosis. Other authors, however, reported a direct correlation between HER2 expression and poorer survival.

Therefore, there is mounting evidence of the role of HER2 overexpression in patients with gastric cancer: HER2 has been solidly correlated to poor outcomes and a more aggressive disease.

Regarding the pathologic variables, a higher rate of HER2 expression in intestinal histologic type than in diffuse type has consistently been reported. GEJ cancer expresses HER2 with more frequency than gastric cancer does.

Several clinical trials are exploring the potential of anti HER2 therapies in gastric cancer patients in different settings and designs.

A high interleukin-1_ (IL-1B) and interleukin-1 receptor antagonist (IL-RN) ratio underlies an unfavorable proinflammatory status. Also, it seems to be involved in the mechanisms of cancer cachexia and tumor angiogenesis and metastasis. Two single nucleotide polymorphisms in *IL-1B* gene (*IL-1B-511C/T,IL-1B-31T/C*) and a variable number of tandem repeat polymorphisms in *IL-RN* gene (*IL-1RNlong/2*) enhance the circulating levels of the two cytokines. Graziano et al. [87] investigated he prognostic role of *IL-1B/IL-1RN* genotypes in patients with relapsed and metastatic gastric cancer treated with palliative chemotherapy. Before starting palliative chemotherapy, 123 prospectively enrolled patients supplied peripheral-blood samples for DNA extraction. Survival data were analyzed according to *IL-1RN/IL-1B* genotypes. Forty-two patients showed wild-type genotypes (*IL-1RNlong/long*, *IL-1B-511C/C*, and *IL-1B-31T/T*; group A). Forty-five patients showed the

IL-1RN2 polymorphism, with wild-type *IL-1B* genotypes in seven patients and with *IL-1B-511C/T* and/or *IL-1B-31T/C* polymorphisms in 38 patients (group B). The remaining 36 patients demonstrated wild-type *IL-1RN*, with *IL-1B-511C/T* and/or *IL-1B-31T/C* polymorphisms (group C). In group A and B patients, the median progression-free survival (PFS) was 25 and 26 weeks, respectively, and median overall survival (OS) was 42 and 43 weeks, respectively. Group C patients showed worse PFS (median, 16 weeks) and OS (median, 28 weeks) than group A (*P* _ .006 for PFS; *P* _ .0001 for OS) and group B patients (*P* _ .01 for PFS; *P* .0001 for OS). The *long/T/C* haplotype was overrepresented in patients with shortened PFS (*P* _ .001) and OS (*P* _ .0005).

Therefore, in patients with advanced gastric cancer *IL-1B* polymorphisms showed adverse prognostic influence when coupled with wild-type *IL-1RN* genotype. These findings deserve further investigation for potential anticancer activity of recombinant *IL-RN*.

Nevertheless, according to other authors [88], the levels of Interleukin seem to correlate with survival in advanced gastrointestinal cancer patients but is not an independent prognostic indicator.

After the results of trastuzumab in patients with *HER2*-positive gastric cancer, there is increasing interest in the development of targeted therapies in this lethal disease. However, the discovery and the optimal use of these selective treatments requires an adequate knowledge of the target and the potential clinical effects from its inhibition. A number of receptors and downstream pathways are known to be aberrantly activated in gastric cancer, and they may represent new treatment targets beyond *HER2* inhibition. HER2, MET and FGFR2 oncogenic driver alterations define distinct molecular segments for targeted therapies in gastric carcinoma [89]. Among them, the MET receptor and its hepatocyte growth factor (HGF) ligand have frequently been found expressed in gastric carcinomas and are associated with a more aggressive phenotype. The activation of the MET/ HGF pathway promotes proliferative and antiapoptotic activities that are common to many growth factors; in particular *MET* activation demonstrated stimulation of cell-cell detachment, migration, and invasiveness.

Mutations in the kinase domain of the *MET* gene amost lack in gastric carcinomas, and its activation has been mostly attributed to gene amplification. Also, Nakajima et al. [90] and Tsugawa et al. [91] found that survival rates of patients with gastric cancer with *MET* amplification are significantly lower than those of patients without amplification.

Graziano et al. [92] investigated whether the prognosis of patients with high-risk gastric cancer may depend on *MET* copy number gain (CNG) or on an activating truncation within a deoxyadenosine tract element (DATE) in the promoter region of the *MET* ligand HGF.

A single-institution cohort of 230 patients with stage II/III gastric cancer was studied. Formalin fixed paraffin-embedded tumor specimens were used for DNA extraction. Quantitative polymerase chain reaction (qPCR) for *MET* CNG and sequencing for *HGF* DATE truncation (_ 25 deoxyadenosine instead of 30) were used. Results were analyzed for association with disease free survival (DFS) and overall survival (OS). To assess the reliability of the qPCR measurement, a random sample of cases was reanalyzed using an alternative assay (fluorescent in situ hybridization [FISH]) with calculation of the intra-correlation coefficient (ICC).

In 216 assessable patients, *MET* CNG five or more copies and homozygous *HGF*-truncated DATE occurred in 21 patients (10%) and 30 patients (13%), respectively. Patients with *MET* CNG five or more copies (*MET*-positive) showed significantly worse prognosis with multivariate hazard ratio (HR) of 3.02 (95% CI, 1.71 to 5.33; *P* _ .001) for DFS and multivariate HR of 2.91 (95% CI, 1.65 to 5.11; *P* _ .001) for OS. The agreement between qPCR and FISH was high, with ICC _ 0.9% (95% CI, 0.81% to 0.95%; the closer the ICC is to 1, the greater is the agreement). *HGF*-truncated DATE did not show relevant prognostic effect.

In this study, qPCR revealed approximately 10% of white patients with gastric cancer harbouring *MET* CNG of five or more copies. This marker was significantly associated with unfavourable prognosis. This information is relevant to the current clinical development of anti-*MET* compounds.

Rilotumumab is a fully human monoclonal antibody (IgG2) against human hepatocyte growth factor/scatter factor (HGF/SF) that blocks binding of HGF/SF to its receptor MET, inhibiting HGF/MET – driven activities in cells.

Phase two studies seem to indicate the overexpression of MET could be a predictor of response to therapy with rilotumumab.

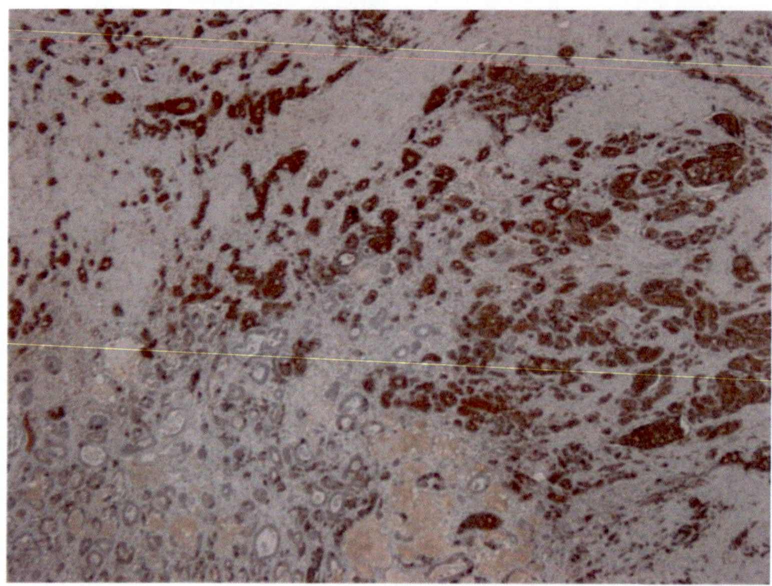

Figure 2. Endocrine differentiation in common gastric cancer (Chromogranin A positivity).

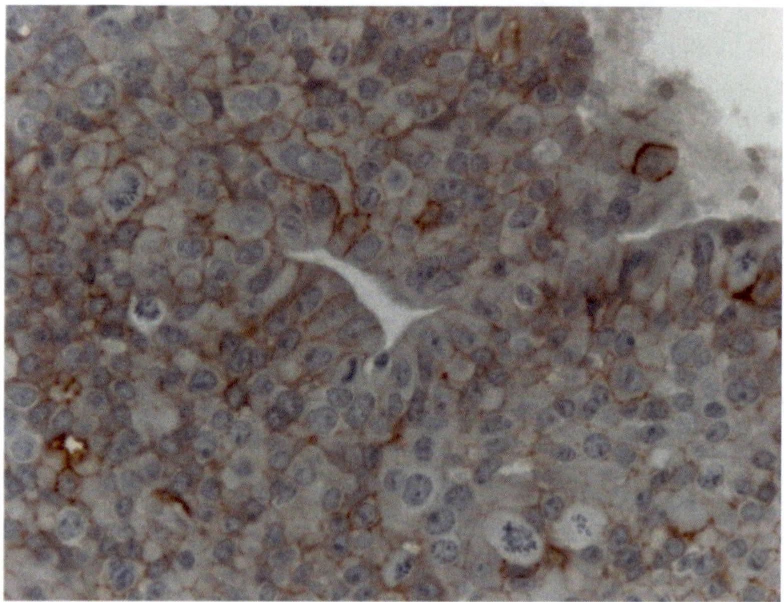

Figure 3. HER2 focal positivity score 3+ in gastric cancer.

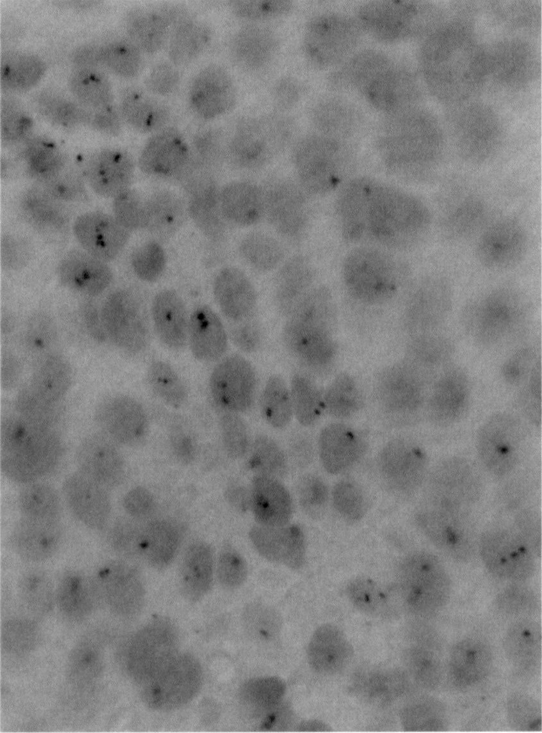

Figure 4. Silver In situ Hybridization (SISH) for the detection of HER 2 amplification in gastric cancer.

Clinical Follow up

Although there is broad agreement in the staging, classification, and surgery for gastric cancer, there is no consensus regarding follow-up after gastrectomy. Follow-up varies from investigations on clinical suspicion of relapse to intensive investigations to detect recurrences early, assuming that this improves survival and quality of life. Advanced gastric cancers recur mainly by locoregional recurrence or distant metastasis [93, 94].

Peritoneum followed by liver metastases are the most frequent distant sites of relapse [95–98].

Local recurrences detected at endoscopy or on computed tomography (CT) are invariably incurable. For early gastric cancers, endoscopy can detect new primaries, but the incidence of these tumors is low, and many thousands of procedures are required to detect each operable case. CT is much better at detecting liver metastasis and, although these are usually multiple and unresectable, there are several reports of good survival following liver resection for isolated metastasis.

Tumor markers have been used with some success to detect subclinical recurrences and could be used to target more invasive or expensive procedures.

There are many investigations that may be used to detect recurrent gastric cancer, and these can broadly be divided into endoscopy, imaging, and blood tests. Endoscopy has the ability to detect intraluminal recurrences with a high degree of accuracy and it also has the ability to detect new cancers at a treatable stage.

The use of tumor markers has become more commonplace. CEA and CA 19-9 levels are easily determined by a simple blood test and have reported sensitivities of between 16% and 65% for individual markers, increasing to up to 85% when both were used in combination. Increases in markers are commonly seen prior to the clinical detection of recurrences, and in a prospective study, both tumor markers were useful indicators of recurrence, even in patients whose original tumors did not express them. Other tumor markers, such CA 125, have been investigated, but sensitivities are significantly lower than those for CEA and CA19-.9.

Reports on the use of imaging in detecting recurrent gastric cancer are few, and are often limited. The ability to detect hepatic metastases is probably also overestimated, and has been examined in a recent meta-analysis of trials comparing the accuracy of several imaging methods. When the required specificity was set at greater than 85%, the most sensitive method was 18F-fluorodeoxyglucose positron emission tomography (PET) with a sensitivity of 90%, followed by magnetic resonance imaging (MRI; 76%), CT (72%), and ultrasonography (US; 55%) [99-102]. In gastric cancer, the great majority of patients under follow-up will not develop hepatic metastases, and even with high specificities, there are likely to be many false-positive results. The ability of CT to primarily diagnose a primary carcinoma of the stomach is not as good as its ability to stage a known cancer, and there is a direct trade-off between sensitivity and specificity.

Therefore, the imaging in the search for asymptomatic recurrence is fraught with difficulties, missing many recurrences and producing a number of false-positive results. Imaging is perhaps more useful when a clinical recurrence is suspected, such as in the face of rising tumormarkers. In this role, PET can be especially useful in cases where conventional imaging results are equivocal, as it can confirm or refute the presence of recurrence in most cases.

References

[1] Jemal, A., Bray, F., Center, M. M., et al. Global cancer statistics. *CA Cancer J. Clin.* 2011; 61:69.

[2] Siegel, R., Naishadham, D., Jemal, A. Cancer statistics, 2013. *CA Cancer J. Clin.* 2013; 63:11.

[3] Parkin, D. M. Epidemiology of cancer: global patterns and trends. *Toxicol. Lett.* 1998; 102-103:227.

[4] Pisani, P., Parkin, D. M., Ferlay, J. Estimates of the worldwide mortality from eighteen major cancers in 1985. Implications for prevention and projections of future burden. *Int. J. Cancer* 1993; 55:891.

[5] Haenszel, W. Variation in incidence of and mortality from stomach cancer, with particular reference to the United States. *J. Natl. Cancer Inist.* 1958; 21:213.

[6] V. Catalano et al., Gastric cancer, *Critical Reviews in Oncology/ Hematology* 71 (2009) 127–164.

[7] Zhu, A. L., Sonnenberg, A. Is gastric cancer again rising? *J. Clin. Gastroenterol.* 2012; 46:804.

[8] Wynder, E. L., Kmet, J., Dungal, N., Segi, M. An epidemiological Investigation of gastric Cancer. *Cancer* 1963; 16:1461.

[9] Correa, P., Haenszel, W., Tannenbaum, S. *Epidemiology of gastric carcinoma: review and future.*

[10] Scheiman, J. M., Cutler, A. F.: Helicobacter pylori and gastric cancer. Am J Med 106 (2): 222-6, 1999. [PUBMED Abstract]rospects. *Natl. Cancer Inst. Monogr.* 1982; 62:129.

[11] Hirayama, T. Epidemiology of cancer of the stomach with special reference to its recent decrease in Japan. *Cancer Res.* 1975; 35:3460.

[12] OPCS (Office of Population, Census and Surveys). *1994 Cancer statistics: Registrations in England and Wales (Series MB No.21).* HMSO, London 1978.

[13] Fitzsimmons, D., Osmond, C., George, S., Johnson, C. D. Trends in stomach and pancreatic cancer incidence and mortality in England and Wales, 1951-2000. *Br. J. Surg.* 2007; 94:1162.

[14] Chen, J. S., Campbell, T. C., Li, J. Y., et al. Life-style and Mortality in China. *A Study of the Characteristics of 65 Chinese Counties*, Oxford University Press, Oxford 1990.

[15] Jemal, A., Siegel, R., Ward, E., et al. Cancer statistics, 2006. *CA Cancer J. Clin.* 2006; 56:106.

[16] Schlansky, B., Sonnenberg, A. Epidemiology of noncardia gastric adenocarcinoma in the United States. *Am. J. Gastroenterol.* 2011; 106: 1978.

[17] Anderson, W. F., Camargo, M. C., Fraumeni, J. F. Jr, et al. Age-specific trends in incidence of noncardia gastric cancer in US adults. *JAMA* 2010; 303:1723.

[18] Coggon, D., Barker, D. J., Cole, R. B., Nelson, M. Stomach cancer and food storage. *J. Natl. Cancer Inst.* 1989; 81:1178.

[19] La Vecchia, C., Negri, E., D'Avanzo, B., Franceschi, S. Electric refrigerator use and gastric cancer risk. *Br. J. Cancer* 1990; 62:136.

[20] Allum, W. H., Powell, D. J., McConkey, C. C., Fielding, J. W. Gastric cancer: a 25-year review. *Br. J. Surg*. 1989;76:535–40.

[21] Wanebo, H. J., Kennedy, B. J., Chmiel, J., et al. Cancer of the stomach. A patient care study by the American College of Surgeons. *Ann. Surg.* 1993;218:583–92.

[22] Akoh, J. A., Macintyre, I. M. Improving survival in gastric cancer: review of 5-year survival rates in English language publications from 1970. *Br. J. Surg*. 1992;79:293–9.

[23] Kurtz, R. C., Sherlock, P.: The diagnosis of gastric cancer. *Semin. Oncol.* 12 (1): 11-8, 1985. [PUBMED Abstract].

[24] Alexander, H. R., Kelsen, D., Tepper, J. C. Cancer of the stomach. In: De Vita, V., Hellman, S., Rosenberg, S., editors. *Cancer: principles and practice of oncology*. 5th edition Philadelphia: JB Lippincott; 1997. p. 1021–54.

[25] Hermanek, P., Maruyama, K., Sobin, L. H. Gastric cancer. In: Hermanek, Gospodarowicz, M. K., Henson, D. E., Hutter, R. V. P., Sobin, L. H., editors. *Prognostic factors in cancer*. Geneve: International Union Against Cancer (UICC); 1995.

[26] Alexander, H. R., Kelsen, D., Tepper, J. C. Cancer of the stomach. In: De Vita, V., Hellman, S., Rosenberg, S., editors. *Cancer: principles and practice of oncology*. 5th edition Philadelphia: JB Lippincott; 1997. p. 1021–54.

[27] UICC (International Union Against Cancer). In: Sobin, L. H., Wittekind, C. H., editors. *TNM classification of malignant tumours*. 5th edition New York, Chichester, Weinheim, Brisbane, Singapore, Toronto: Wiley-Liss; 1997.

[28] van Krieken, J. H., Sasako, M., van de velde, C. J. Gastric cancer. In: Gospodarowicz, M. K., Henson, D. E., Hutter, R. V. P., O'Sullivan, B.,

Sobin, L. H., Wittekind, C., editors. *Prognostic factors in cancer*. New York: Wiley-Liss; 2001. p. 251–65.

[29] Rohde, H., Gebbensleben, B., Bauer, P., Stutzer, H., Zieschang, J. Has there been any improvement in the staging of gastric cancer? Findings from the German Gastric Cancer TNM Study Group. *Cancer* 1989;64: 2465–81.

[30] Carriaga, M. T., Henson, D. E. The histologic grading of cancer. *Cancer* 1995;75:406–21.

[31] Lauren, P. The two histological main types of Gastric Carcinoma: Diffuse and so-called intestinal-type carcinoma. An attempt at a histo-clinical classification. *Acta Pathol. Microbiol. Scand.* 1965; 64:31.

[32] Ikeda, Y., Mori, M., Kamakura, T., et al. Improvements in diagnosis have changed the incidence of histological types in advanced gastric cancer. *Br. J. Cancer* 1995; 72:424.

[33] *J. Clin. Oncol.* 2012 Oct. 1;30(28):3493-8. Epub. 2012 Aug. 27. Prognostic significance of signet ring gastric cancer. Taghavi S1, Jayarajan SN, Davey A, Willis AI.

[34] Bunt, A. M., Hogendoorn, P. C., van de Velde, C. J., Bruijn, J. A., Hermans, J. Lymph node staging standards in gastric cancer. *J. Clin. Oncol.* 1995;13:2309–16.

[35] Hartgrink, H. H., Bonenkamp, H. J., van de Velde, C. J. Influence of surgery on outcomes in gastric cancer. *Surg. Oncol. Clin. N. Am.* 2000;9: 91–117.

[36] Siewert, J. R., Bottcher, K., Stein, H. J., Roder, J. D. Relevant prognostic factors in gastric cancer: ten-year results of the German Gastric Cancer Study. *Ann. Surg.* 1998;228:449–61.

[37] British Stomach Cancer Group. Resection line disease in stomach cancer. *Br. Med. J.* (Clin. Res. Ed.) 1984;289:601–3.

[38] Fujimoto, S., Takahashi, M., Mutou, T., et al. Clinicopathologic characteristics of gastric cancer patients with cancer infiltration at surgical margin at gastrectomy. *Anticancer Res.* 1997;17:689–94.

[39] Takagane, A., Terashima, M., Abe, K., et al. Evaluation of the ratio of lymph node metastasis as a prognostic factor in patients with gastric cancer. *Gastric Cancer* 1999;2:122–8.

[40] Bollschweiler, E., Boettcher, K., Hoelscher, A. H., et al. Is the prognosis for Japanese and German patients with gastric cancer really different? *Cancer* 1993;71:2918–25.

[41] Maehara, Y., Kakeji, Y., Oda, S., et al. Time trends of surgical treatment and the prognosis for Japanese patients with gastric cancer. *Br. J. Cancer* 2000;83:986–91.

[42] Moriguchi, S., Maehara, Y., Korenaga, D., Sugimachi, K., Nose, Y. Relationship between age and the time of surgery and prognosis after gastrectomy for gastric cancer. *J. Surg. Oncol.* 1993;52:119–23.

[43] Maguire, A., Porta, M., Sanz-Anquela, J. M., et al. Sex as a prognostic factor in gastric cancer. *Eur. J. Cancer* 1996;32A:1303–9.

[44] Maehara, Y., Watanabe, A., Kakeji, Y., et al. Prognosis for surgically treated gastric cancer patients is poorer for women than men in all patients under age 50. *Br. J. Cancer* 1992;65:417–20.

[45] *World J. Surg.* 2004 Feb.; 28(2):155-9. Epub. 2004 Jan. 8. Presentation and prognosis of gastric cancer in patients aged 80 years and older. Rabuñal, R. R. 1., Pita, S. F., Rigueiro, M. T., Casariego, E. V., Pértega, S. D., García-Rodeja, E., Abraira, V.

[46] Tachibana, M., Takemoto, Y., Nakashima, Y., et al. Serum carcinoembryonic antigen as a prognostic factor in resectable gastric cancer. *J. Am. Coll. Surg.* 1998;187:64–8.

[47] Nakane, Y., Okamura, S., Akehira, K., et al. Correlation of preoperative carcinoembryonic antigen levels and prognosis of gastric cancer patients. *Cancer* 1994;73:2703–8.

[48] Sakamoto, J., Nakazato, H., Teramukai, S., et al. Association between preoperative plasma CEA levels and the prognosis of gastric cancer following curative resection. Tumor Marker Committee, Japanese Foundation for Multidisciplinary Treatment of Cancer, Tokyo, Japan. *Surg. Oncol.* 1996;5:133–9.

[49] Maehara, Y., Kusumoto, T., Takahashi, I., et al. Predictive value of preoperative carcinoembryonic antigen levels for the prognosis of patients with well-differentiated gastric cancer. A multivariate analysis. *Oncology* 1994;51:234–7.

[50] Irinoda, T., Terashima, M., Takagane, A., et al. Carcinoembryonic antigen level in peritoneal washing is a prognostic factor in patients with gastric cancer. *Oncol. Rep.* 1998;5:661–6.

[51] Nishiyama, M., Takashima, I., Tanaka, T., et al. Carcinoembryonic antigen levels in the peritoneal cavity: useful guide to peritoneal recurrence and prognosis for gastric cancer. *World J. Surg.* 1995;19: 133–7.

[52] J. Chung et al., Comparison of the validity of three biomarkers for gastric cancer screening: carcinoembryonic antigen, pepsinogens, and high sensitive C-reactive protein. *Clin. Gastroenterol.* 2009 Jan.;43(1): 19-26. doi: 10.1097/MCG.0b013e318135427c.

[53] Kodama et al., The clinical efficacy of CA 72-4 as serum marker for gastric cancer in comparison with CA19-9 and CEA. *Int. Surg.* 1995 Jan.-Mar.;80(1):45-8.

[54] Ucar et al., Prognostic value of preoperative CEA, CA 19-9, CA 72-4, and AFP levels in gastric cancer. *Adv. Ther.* 2008 Oct.;25(10):1075-84. doi: 10.1007/s12325-008-0100-4.

[55] Nakanishi et al., Rapid quantitative detection of carcinoembryonic antigen-expressing free tumor cells in the peritoneal cavity of gastric-cancer patients with real-time RT-PCR on the lightcycler, *Int. J. Cancer.* 2000 Sep. 20;89(5):411-7.

[56] Mattar et al., Preoperative serum levels of CA 72-4, CEA, CA 19-9, and alpha-fetoprotein in patients with gastric cancer. *Rev. Hosp. Clin. Fac. Med. Sao Paulo.* 2002 May-Jun.;57(3):89-92.

[57] Fernandes et al., CA72-4 antigen levels in serum and peritoneal washing in gastric cancer. Correlation with morphological aspects of neoplasia, *Arq. Gastroenterol.* 2007 Jul.-Sep.;44(3):235-9.

[58] Becker, K. F., Keller, G., Hoefler, H. The use of molecular biology in diagnosis and prognosis of gastric cancer. *Surg. Oncol.* 2000;9: 5–11.

[59] Fenoglio-Preiser, C. M., Wang, J., Stemmermann, G. N., Noffsinger, A. TP53 and gastric carcinoma: a review. *Hum. Mutat.* 2003;21: 258–70.

[60] Tahara, E., Semba, S., Tahara, H. Molecular biological observations in gastric cancer. *Semin. Oncol.* 1996;23:307–15.

[61] Kubicka, S., Claas, C., Staab, S., et al. p53 mutation pattern and expression of c-erbB2 and c-met in gastric cancer: relation to histological subtypes, helicobacter pylori infection, and prognosis. *Dig. Dis. Sci.* 2002;47:114–21.

[62] Maeda, K., Kang, S. M., Onoda, N., et al. Expression of p53 and vascular endothelial growth factor associated with tumor angiogenesis and prognosis in gastric cancer. *Oncology* 1998;55:594–9.

[63] Fonseca, L., Yonemura, Y., De, A. X., et al. p53 detection as a prognostic factor in early gastric cancer. *Oncology* 1994;51:485–90.

[64] Victorzon, M., Nordling, S., Haglund, C., Lundin, J., Roberts, P. J. Expression of p53 protein as a prognostic factor in patients with gastric cancer. *Eur. J. Cancer* 1996;32A:215–20.

[65] Xiangming, C., Hokita, S., Natsugoe, S., et al. p21 expression is a prognostic factor in patients with p53-negative gastric cancer. *Cancer Lett.*, 2000;148:181–8.

[66] Catalano, V., Baldelli, A. M., Giordani, P., Cascinu, S. Molecular markers predictive of response to chemotherapy in gastrointestinal tumors. *Crit. Rev. Oncol. Hematol.* 2001;38:93–104.

[67] Cascinu, S., Graziano, F., Del Ferro, E., et al. Expression of p53 protein protein and resistance to preoperative chemotherapy in locally advanced gastric carcinoma. *Cancer* 1998;83:1917–22.

[68] Nakata, B., Chung, K. H., Ogawa, M., et al. p53 protein overexpression as a predictor of the response to chemotherapy in gastric cancer. *Surg. Today* 1998;28:595–8.

[69] Lenz, H. J., Leichman, C. G., Danenberg, K. D., et al. Thymidylate synthase mRNA level in adenocarcinoma of the stomach: a predictor for primary tumor response and overall survival. *J. Clin. Oncol.* 1996;14: 176–82.

[70] Yeh, K. H., Shun, C. T., Chen, C. L., et al. High expression of thymidylate synthase is associated with the drug resistance of gastric carcinoma to high dose 5-fluorouracil-based systemic chemotherapy. *Cancer* 1998;82:1626–31.

[71] Metzger, R., Leichman, C. G., Danenberg, K. D., et al. ERCC1 mRNA levels complement thymidylate synthase mRNA levels in predicting response and survival for gastric cancer patients receiving combination cisplatin and fluorouracil chemotherapy. *J. Clin. Oncol.* 1998;16:309–16.

[72] Annie On-On Chan et al., Soluble E-Cadherin is an Independent Pretherapeutic Factor for Long-Term Survival in Gastric Cancer – JCO 2003.

[73] Frixen, U. H., Behrens, J., Sachs, M., et al.: E-cadherin-mediated cell-cell adhesion prevents invasiveness of human carcinoma cells. *J. Cell Biol.* 113:173-185, 1991.

[74] Vleminckx, K., Vakaet, L. Jr, Mareel, M., et al.: Genetic manipulation of E-cadherin expression by epithelial tumor cells reveals an invasion suppressor role. *Cell* 66:107-119, 1991.

[75] Canzonieri, V.(1), Colarossi, C., Del Col, L., Perin, T., Talamini, R., Sigon, R., Cannizzaro, R., Aiello, E., Buonadonna, A., Italia, F., Massi, D., Carbone, A., Memeo, L. Exocrine and endocrine modulation in common gastric carcinoma. *Am. J. Clin. Pathol.* 2012 May;137(5):712-21.

[76] Kang, Y., Bang, Y., Lordick, F., et al. Incidence of gastric and gastro-esophageal cancer in the ToGA trial: correlation with HER2 positivity. *2008 Gastrointestinal Cancers Symposium*. 75 (Abstr. 11).

[77] Tateishi, M., Toda, T., Minamisono, Y., et al. Clinicopathological significance of c-erbB-2 protein expression in human gastric carcinoma. *Surg. Oncol.* 1992; 49:209–212.

[78] Sasano, H., Date, F., Imatani, A., et al. Double immunostaining for c-erbB-2 and p53 in human stomach cancer cells. *Hum. Pathol.* 1993; 24: 584–589.

[79] Uchino, S., Tsuda, H., Maruyama, K., et al. Overexpression of c-erbB-2 protein in gastric cancer. Its correlation with long-term survival of patients. *Cancer* 1993.

[80] Mizutani, T., Onda, M., Tokunaga, A., et al. Relationship of c-erbB-2 protein expression and gene amplification to invasion and metastasis in human gastric cancer. *Cancer* 1993; 72: 2083–2088.

[81] Garcia, I., Vizoso, F., Martin, A., et al. Clinical significance of the epidermal growth factor receptor and HER2 receptor in resectable gastric cancer. *Ann. Surg. Oncol.* 2003; 10(3): 234–241.

[82] Tanner, M., Hollmen, M., Junttila, T. T., et al. Amplification of HER-2 in gastric carcinoma: association with topoisomerase IIa gene amplification, intestinal type, poor prognosis and sensitivity to trastuzumab. *Ann. Oncol.* 2005; 16: 273–278.

[83] Takehana, T., Kunimoto, K., Kono, K., et al. Status of c-erbB-2 in gastric adenocarcinoma: a comparative study of immunohistochemistry, fluorescence in situ hybridization and enzyme-linked immuno-sorbent assay. *Int. J. Cancer* 2002; 98: 833–837.

[84] Lin, J. T., Wu, M. S., Shun, C. T., et al. Occurrence of microsatellite instability in gastric carcinoma is associated with enhanced expression of erbB-2 oncoprotein. *Cancer Res.* 1995; 55: 1428–1430.

[85] HER2 in gastric cancer: a new prognostic factor and a novel therapeutic target. *Annals of Oncology* 19: 1523–1529, 2008.

[86] Bang, Y. J., et al., Trastuzumab in combination with chemotherapy versus chemotherapy alone for treatment of HER2-positive advanced gastric or gastro-oesophageal junction cancer (ToGA): a phase 3, open-label, randomised controlled trial, *Lancet.* 2010 Aug. 28;376(9742):687-97. doi: 10.1016/S0140-6736(10)61121-X. Epub. 2010 Aug. 19. Erratum in: *Lancet.* 2010 Oct. 16;376(9749):1302.

[87] Graziano et al., Prognostic Role of Interleukin-1Gene and Interleukin-1 Receptor Antagonist Gene Polymorphisms in Patients With Advanced Gastric Cancer, *J. Clin. Oncol.* 2005 Apr. 1;23(10):2339-45.

[88] De Vita, F., et al., Interleukin-6 serum level correlates with survival in advanced gastrointestinal cancer patients but is not an independent prognostic indicator, *J. Interferon Cytokine Res.* 2001 Jan.;21(1):45-52.

[89] Liu, Y. J., et al., HER2, MET and FGFR2 oncogenic driver alterations define distinct molecular segments for targeted therapies in gastric carcinoma, *Br. J. Cancer.* 2014 Feb 11. doi: 10.1038/bjc.2014.61. [Epub. ahead of print].

[90] Nakajima, M., et al., The prognostic significance of amplification and overexpression of c-met and c-erb B-2 in human gastric carcinomas, *Cancer.* 1999 May 1;85(9):1894-902.

[91] Tsugawa, K. et al., Amplification of the c-met, c-erbB-2 and epidermal growth factor receptor gene in human gastric cancers: correlation to clinical features, *Oncology.* 1998 Sep.-Oct.;55(5):475-81.

[92] Graziano et al., Genetic Activation of the MET Pathway and Prognosis of Patients With High-Risk, *Radically Resected Gastric Cancer, JCO* 2011.

[93] Wu, C. W., Lo, S. S., Shen, K. H., et al. Incidence and factors associated with recurrence patterns after intended curative surgery for gastric cancer. *World J. Surg.* 2003;27:153–8.

[94] Shiraishi, N., Inomata, M., Osawa, N., et al. Early and late recurrence after gastrectomy for gastric carcinoma, Univariate and multivariate analyses. *Cancer* 2000;89:255–61.

[95] Wu, C. W., Lo, S. S., Shen, K. H., et al. Incidence and factors associated with recurrence patterns after intended curative surgery for gastric cancer. *World J. Surg.* 2003;27:153–8.

[96] Shiraishi, N., Inomata, M., Osawa, N., et al. Early and late recurrence after gastrectomy for gastric carcinoma, Univariate and multivariate analyses. *Cancer* 2000;89:255–61.

[97] Landry, J., Tepper, J. E., Wood, W. C., et al. Patterns of failure following curative resection of gastric carcinoma. *Int. J. Radiat. Oncol. Biol. Phys.* 1990;19:1357–62.

[98] Katai, H., Maruyama, K., Sasako, M., et al. Mode of recurrence after gastric cancer surgery. *Dig. Surg.* 1994;11:99–103.

[99] Małkowski, B., et al., (18)F-FLT PET/CT in Patients with Gastric Carcinoma, *Gastroenterol. Res. Pract.* 2013;2013:696423. doi: 10.1155/ 2013/696423. Epub. 2013 Dec. 25.

[100] Lacueva, F. J., Calpena, R., Medrano, J., et al. Follow-up of patients resected for gastric cancer. *J. Surg. Oncol.* 1995;60:174–9.

[101] Huguier, M., Houry, S., Lacaine, F. Is the follow-up of patients operated on for gastric carcinoma of benefit to the patient? *Hepato-gastroenterology* 1992;39:14–6.

[102] Bohner, H., Zimmer, T., Hopfenmuller, W., Berger, G., Buhr, H. J. Detection and prognosis of recurrent gastric cancer–is routine follow-up after gastrectomy worthwhile? *Hepatogastroenterology* 2000;47:1489–94.

In: Prognostic and Predictive Response ... ISBN: 978-1-63463-545-5
Editors: V. Canzonieri and M. Berretta

Chapter 4

Primary Liver Cancer: Prognostic Factors and Predictive Response to Therapy

A. Valdegamberi, A. Ruzzenente, S. Conci, F. Bagante, A. Cappellani and A. Guglielmi*

Department of Surgery, Division of General Surgery A,
University of Verona Medical School, Verona, Italy

Abstract

Primary liver cancer (PLC) is the fifth most common cancer in men and the seventh most common cancer in women. Up to 85% of cases occur in developing countries. Liver cancer is associated with a high mortality rate that is similar across various geographic regions. Hepatocellular carcinoma (HCC) accounts for up to 85% of all PLC cases. Usually HCC is a consequence of cirrhosis, but it can also develop in the absence of chronic hepatic disease in approximately 20% of patients, especially among those with more severe forms of non-alcoholic fatty liver disease (NAFLD). Currently, both Western and Eastern guidelines recommend only radiological diagnosis in patients with cirrhosis. The most widely accepted system is the Barcelona Clinic Liver Cancer (BCLC) staging system, which was updated in 2011 and was validated by several groups in Western countries. The BCLC staging

* Corresponding author. Policlinico G.B. Rossi lotto I, Floor Piano 3°, Room , University of Verona; Tel +39 0458124464; Fax +39 0458027426 ; email: alfredo.guglielmi@univr.it.

system includes factors of both tumor morphology and degree of impairment of liver function, and it can be used to assign the proper treatment to patients with HCC. However, these treatment allocations have been criticized due to the exclusion from surgical resection of some patients who could potentially benefit from this type of therapy. The treatment of HCC varies in relation to the tumor stage and the degree of hepatic dysfunction. Liver transplantation and surgical resection with radical intent enables good long-term survival and excellent 5-year survival rates (70-50%). In addition, locoregional treatment can also achieve positive results, especially treatment of early-stage nodules.

Intrahepatic cholangiocarcinoma (ICC), the second most common primary liver cancer after HCC, arises from the bile ducts of the second-order and usually presents as a mass inside the liver. CT and MRI imaging are the most useful imaging modalities for the diagnosis of ICC: imaging techniques show the location of the tumor, the possible multifocality of the lesion, the presence of venous or arterial invasion, and the presence of lymphnode involvement or distant metastases. According to the type of macroscopic growth, three types of ICC are described: mass forming (MF), periductal infiltrating (PI), and intraductal growing (IG). Radical surgical resection (R0) is the treatment of choice and the only one able to achieve long-term survival. In order to achieve radical resection, a major hepatectomy is often required, but this therapeutic option still has acceptable mortality and morbidity rates.

Other PLCs (e.g., fibrolamellar hepatocellular carcinoma, epithelioid hemangioendothelioma, hepatoblastoma, sarcoma and lymphomas, combined HCC and ICC) are very rare, and surgery is the treatment of choice for these types of PLCs.

Introduction

Worldwide, primary liver cancer (PLC) is the fifth most common cancer in men and the seventh most common cancer in women. Up to 85% of PLC occurs in developing countries [1]. The rates are highest in Eastern and South-Eastern Asia and Middle and Western Africa but are generally low in developed countries, especially in North America and Europe [2]. In 2008, an estimated 694,000 deaths from liver cancer (477,000 men and 217,000 women) were reported. Liver cancer is associated with a high mortality rate [1] that is similar regardless of geographic region. In 2002, more than 377,000 people died from liver cancer in Eastern Asia, which accounted for 19% of the total number of cancer-related deaths [3].

Here, we consider the clinical and pathological characteristics of hepatocellular carcinoma and cholangiocarcinoma from the prognostic and predictive viewpoints.

Clinical Prognostic Factors of Hepatocellular Carcinoma (HCC)

HCC is the most common PLC and accounts for up to 85% of all PLC cases. It is the sixth most common cancer and the third most frequent cause of cancer-related death. The incidence increases with advancing age, with a median age at onset of approximately 70 years in developed countries. HCC also predominantly affects males and has a male to female ratio of approximately 2.4 [4]. Usually, HCC is a consequence of cirrhosis caused by chronic viral hepatitis C and B, alcoholic hepatitis, autoimmune hepatitis, hemochromatosis, alpha-1-antitrypsin deficiency and Wilson's disease [5]. Nevertheless, it develops in the absence of chronic hepatic disease in approximately 20% of patients. Overall, the incidence of HCC is increasing, not only in patients with cirrhosis[6] but also in some subgroups of patients such as those with human immunodeficiency virus (HIV) infection [7]. Emerging clinical evidence suggests that HCC is one of the most important causes of death among patients with more severe forms of non-alcoholic fatty liver disease (NAFLD). NAFLD encompasses variable degrees of liver damage: steatosis without inflammation (fatty liver), nonalcoholic steatohepatitis (NASH) and cirrhosis [8]. Approximately 20 to 30% of adults of the general population in Western countries have NAFLD, and its prevalence increases to 70-90% among persons who are obese or who have type 2 diabetes [8]. If confirmed in large-scale prospective studies, the potential adverse impact of NAFLD on the development of cirrhosis and HCC will deserve particular attention, especially with respect to the possible implications for screening and surveillance strategies in the growing number of patients with metabolic syndrome (MS) and NAFLD.

Diagnosis

Although in the past the histological-proven biopsy was the gold standard for the diagnosis of HCC, current guidelines recommend a diagnosis solely on the basis of radiological criteria in patients [9-11] with cirrhosis. The commonly accepted criteria for the diagnosis of HCC are contrast enhancement (wash-in) in the arterial phase and wash-out in the venous/late phase, which is referred to as the "wash-in wash-out pattern"(Figure 1). In Western countries, the guidelines that are most frequently applied in clinical practice for diagnosis are those of the American Association for the Study of Liver Disease (AASLD) and the European Association for the Study of the Liver (EASL) [11]. In both sets of guidelines, hepatic nodules more than 2 cm in size with a "wash-in wash-out pattern" in one of the imaging techniques (CT or MRI) indicate a diagnosis of HCC. However, for nodules between 1 and 2 cm, EASL guidelines advise that the typical pattern that is observed in two imaging techniques should agree. Biopsy of the nodules is recommended by both the AASLD and the EASL in the absence of a wash-in wash-out pattern. Remarkably, neither contrast-enhanced ultrasound nor levels of serum alpha-fetoprotein are considered in the diagnostic criteria by either set of guidelines. In Japan, the most widely accepted guidelines are those of the Japanese Society of Hepatology (JSH), which were updated in 2012 [10]. The diagnostic criteria of these guidelines are the wash-in wash-out pattern observed in one type of imaging modality (CT, MR, and even contrast-enhanced ultrasound), an AFP serum value more than 200 ng/dL, a PIVKA-II serum value more than 40 ng/dL, or AFP L3 > 15%.

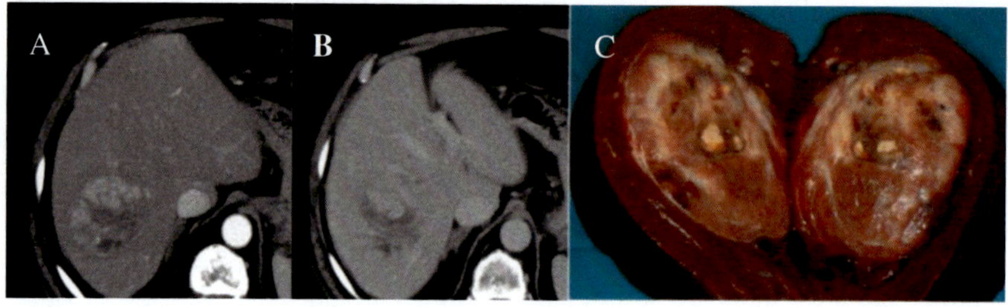

Figure 1. CT scan showing a hepatic nodule with a "wash-in wash-out pattern", diagnosed as HCC. A:Arterial phase. B: venous phase. C: surgical specimen confirmed the diagnosis.

Staging Systems

The importance of staging systems in HCC has been emphasized by several consensus conferences and clinical guidelines. In the literature, the identification of the best staging system for HCC in patients with cirrhosis is still debated due to the relationship between neoplasms and chronic liver disease. Many staging systems have been proposed in the last 20 years, but no convincing evidence has suggested that one system is better than the others. Furthermore, the predictive value of each system is greatly influenced by the characteristics of the cohort of patients enrolled and by the type of treatment that is utilized. Currently, the most accepted system is the Barcelona Clinic Liver Cancer (BCLC) staging system, which was updated in 2011 [9]. The BCLC system was validated by several groups in Europe and the United States and showed good performance in surgical and nonsurgical patients [12-16]. The BCLC staging system includes factors of both tumor morphology and degree of impairment of liver function, and it can be used to assign the proper treatment to patients with HCC, according to their liver function, the PS, and the tumor stage. Recently, this treatment allocation has been carefully criticized by several authors[17, 18] due to the exclusion from surgical resection of patients who might potentially benefit from this type of therapy, such as patients with macroscopic vascular involvement [19]. The TNM system of the International Union Against Cancer (UICC) and American Joint Committee on Cancer (AJCC) [20] is a popular system for use in surgical patients, but controversy persists about its value in HCC due to the absence of variables related to liver function. Furthermore, clinical studies have shown non-homogeneous stratification of risks among individuals of different stages due to the defined criteria of the T-stage. The system proposed by the Cancer of the Liver Italian Program (CLIP) [21] in 1998 was based on a retrospective study of 435 patients with HCC. The CLIP identified five independent variables: Child-Pugh class, tumor size, number of tumors, presence of portal thrombosis, and serum AFP. The validity of this system was confirmed by large validation studies in Italy, Canada, and Japan [22, 23]. The greatest criticism of the CLIP classification is that it includes a large set of advanced stage morphologic criteria, which reduces its value in patients with early-stage HCC. The Japan Integrated Staging score (JIS) [24]was proposed in 2003 as the combination of the Child-Pugh score for liver function and the modified TNM classification according to the Liver Cancer Study Group of Japan (LCSGJ). The JIS score was validated by a statistical analysis of patients after surgical resection of HCC, but this system has not been validated in other cohorts of patients who were treated with nonsurgical modes of therapy.

Management of HCC

The treatment of HCC varies in relation to the tumor stage and the degree of hepatic dysfunction. Classically, the best survival results have been reported when the following indications were satisfied: single tumors and good liver function (no portal hypertension, normal bilirubin) for resection, single tumors ≤5 cm or three nodules ≤3 cm for liver transplantation, and single tumors ≤3 cm in Child-Pugh A patients for percutaneous treatments [25]. Following these indications, a survival of 50–70% at 5 years can be achieved [25].

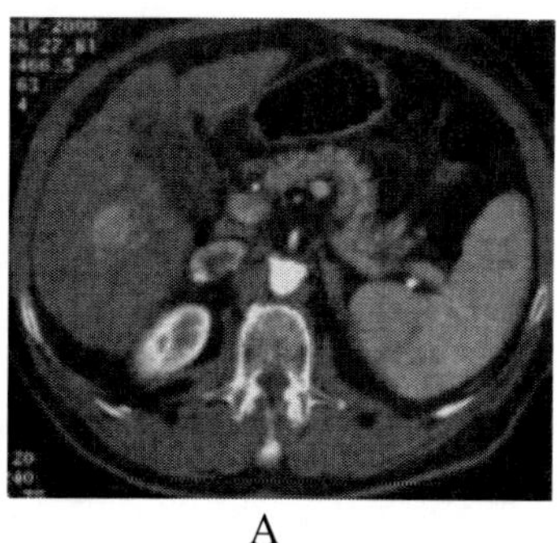

A

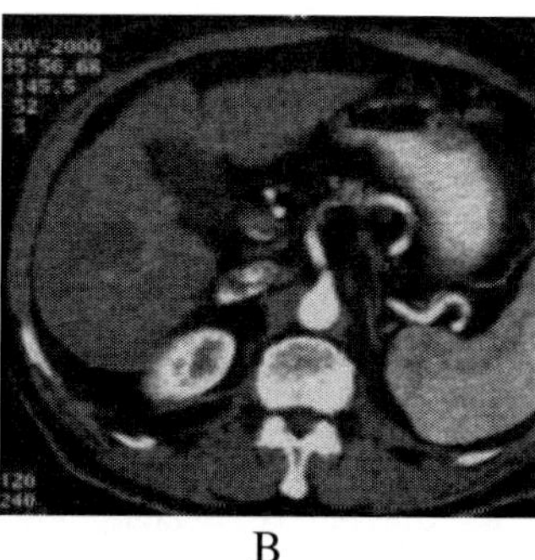

B

Figure 2. A: CT scan in the arterial phase showing HCC nodules 23 mm in size. B: A hypodense nodule in the control CT scan demonstrated a complete response after radiofrequency ablation.

Early HCC

When applied during early stages of the disease, liver transplantation enables an excellent 5-year survival (70-75%) and is associated with low rates of recurrence (10-15%) [26]. Unfortunately, because of the shortage of organs and the strict selection criteria, this resource is confined to only a few patients. In contrast, surgical resection is applicable to approximately 20-30% of patients. Surgical resection is safe and is associated with low rates of mortality (0-3%) and morbidity (25-30%). In patients with moderate liver impairment, resection requires a careful preoperative assessment of liver function with biochemical and dynamic parameters, such as the indocyanine green retention test [27]. Surgical resection with radical intent enables good long-term survival: 40-50% at 5 years [17]. In HCCs smaller than 3 cm, the 5-year survival exceeds 60%, with a 10-year survival of 20% [28]. Until a few years ago, the presence of portal hypertension was considered an absolute contraindication to surgical resection. However, recent data show that in patients with moderate portal hypertension who were classified as Child-Pugh class A limited (up to two segments), liver resection can be performed with results that are comparable to those of patients without portal hypertension [17]. According to the data in the literature, in patients with small HCCs (less than 2 cm in size), percutaneous local treatments (e.g., radiofrequency ablation) offer good long-term results that are comparable to the results after surgery [29]. These data were confirmed by a recent review of the literature in which the authors concluded that it is reasonable to offer radiofrequency ablation to patients with HCCs less than 2 cm in size. On the contrary, for larger nodules or in tumor locations in which ablation is not expected to be effective or safe, surgical removal is preferred [30] (Figure 2).

Intermediate-advanced HCCA

Approximately 20% of patients with HCC are classified as intermediate-stage HCC. The expected 2-year survival rate is 50% [31]. Intermediate-stage HCC includes a heterogeneous population of patients with different tumor burden, liver function and disease etiology [32, 33]. Patients in an intermediate stage (i.e., large and/or multinodular HCC in asymptomatic patients without a neoplastic vascular invasion) showed a 3-year survival rate of 50% compared with patients at a more advanced stage, who showed a 3-year survival rate of 8% [34]. Resection may still be a valid option in selected patients [35]. Radical resection can be considered in patients with large single HCC nodules with well-compensated liver function and adequate remnant liver volume and in selected patients with multinodular HCC or in patients with limited macroscopic vascular invasion; the 5-year survival is 46% in patients with multifocal HCC and is 20% in patients with macroscopic vascular invasion [19, 35]. Nevertheless, transarterial chemoembolization (TACE), particularly selective or superselective TACE, is considered the standard treatment of patients with compensated liver function (Child-Pugh A and Child B up to 7 points), with large single nodules (<5 cm) or multifocal HCC that does not occluding the portal venous vessels and in those without extrahepatic spread [35]. The literature has reported survival benefits of TACE when compared to symptomatic treatment, with a 2-year survival rate of 30% [36]. TACE-associated adverse events, although usually transient and manageable, occur in a significant proportion (35–90%) of patients: they include post-embolization syndrome (fever, abdominal pain), relevant liver function deterioration, ascites and gastrointestinal bleeding [36]. Selective/superselective TACE may determine a higher rate of tumor necrosis than the standard TACE, with fewer reported adverse events [37].

Radioembolization is a form of brachytherapy in which intra-arterially injected radioactive microspheres loaded with yttrium 90 (^{90}Y) are used for internal radiation purposes. Its aim is to deliver tumoricidal doses of radiation to liver tumors while sparing the normal liver. All of the evidence that supports the use of radioembolization in cases of HCC is based on retrospective series or non-controlled prospective studies, but some evidence has been provided that radioembolization can prolong survival over non-specific therapy in patients who are not amenable to TACE. This evidence is further supported by the comparison of numerous studies that have reported survival rates in the range of 9–16 months [38].

Medical Treatment

Sorafenib is an oral molecular-targeted multi-kinase inhibitor of the vascular endothelial growth factor receptor and the platelet-derived growth factor receptor. It is the only chemotherapeutic agent that has demonstrated a significant improvement in the time to progression and in the overall survival of patients with advanced HCC. The adverse effects are easily managed without treatment-related mortality [39, 40]. Its use is recommended for patients with HCC who demonstrate good performance status (PS) and Child-Pugh class A advanced HCC and patients for whom other treatments are not indicated [41]. The reported median overall survival in these patients is 10.7 months [40].

End-stage HCC

Patients with end-stage disease present as Okuda stage III or with a Performance Status of 3–4 that reflects a severe tumor-related disability. Similarly, patients with tumors with a Child-Pugh score of C also account for a very poor prognosis. The 6-month survival rate in these patients is 5% [5].

Recurrence

Recurrence of HCC is the major drawback of potentially curative treatments. Even after curative resection, recurrence is very frequent and occurs in approximately 70-100% of cases within 5 years of treatment [42]. Recurrence can be due to the presence of intrahepatic metastases or to neocarcinogenesis in the remnant liver. In the literature, many prognostic factors related to recurrence have been identified, and among these, the most important are the size, the absence of a pseudocapsule, the presence of satellite nodules, vascular invasion, tumor grading and the serum levels of alpha-fetoprotein [43]. The activity of the underlying liver disease, the type of viral infection and the degree of fibrosis are related to the development of recurrence secondary to neocarcinogenesis [44]. New molecular markers that are related to early recurrence have recently been proposed, which may help with the understanding of the biological subclasses and the optimization of benefits from molecular therapies. Actually, no molecular classification has demonstrated its ability to precisely predict survival and recurrence of HCC in a clinical setting. A recent study seemed to prove that *C-MYC* status is an important prognostic factor: the amplified *C-MYC* status was associated with a risk of recurrence that is significantly higher compared to disomic and polysomic status. Additionally, for OS, amplified *C-MYC* status was the strongest prognostic factor in both univariate and multivariate analyses [45].

Intrahepatic Cholangiocarcinoma (ICC)

Intrahepatic cholangiocarcinoma (ICC) is the second most common primary liver cancer after HCC, and it accounts for 3% of all gastrointestinal cancers. Because it arises from the epithelial cells of the bile duct, the most common histologic type is adenocarcinoma [46]. Intrahepatic cholangiocarcinoma arises from the bile ducts of the second order and usually presents as a mass inside the liver [47]. Patients typically present in the sixth and seventh decades of life. According to evidence from autoptic studies, the prevalence of the ICC is estimated to be between 0.01% and 0.5%. The incidence and mortality of ICC are increasing worldwide, both in industrialized and developing countries. The incidence registered in the U.S. is 1-2 cases per 100,000 inhabitants, with 3,500 new cases each year[48, 49]. The highest rates of incidence are in Southeast Asia (Thailand, Cambodia, Laos), which is due to the greater prevalence of risk factors [50] such as the following: congenital anomalies of the biliary tract, congenital cysts of the biliary tree, primary sclerosing cholangitis, hepatolithiasis, liver fluke infections, bile duct adenoma, and environmental toxins (e.g., tobacco, dioxin, vinyl chloride) [48]. Based on the type of macroscopic growth, three types of ICC are described: mass forming (MF), periductal infiltrating (PI), and intraductal growing (IG). The MF type presents as a nodular growth with a well-defined margin, while the PI type presents as a diffuse infiltrative growth along the axis of the portal tracts without a clearly defined mass. The IG type manifests as a papillary growth inside of a bile duct. Mixed forms are classified by the specification of the most represented macroscopic features (i.e., type MF + PI) [51].

Diagnosis

ICC occurs frequently without specific symptoms, such as tenderness in the abdomen, weight loss, malaise and anorexia. In some cases, the only finding is an abdominal mass that can be detected during radiological examinations. The laboratory tests show moderately elevated levels of alkaline phosphatase, gamma-glutamyl transferase and bilirubin in the serum. Increases in CA 19.9 levels can be seen in as many as 85% of patients. The serum levels of CEA (in 30% of cases) and CA 125 (in 40-50% of patients) can also be elevated. Bile duct obstruction, if present, can cause an increase in prothrombin time and a reduction in fat-soluble vitamins. Advanced stages could show an impaired hepatic function due to the replacement of the liver parenchyma by the tumor [52]. Abdominal ultrasound is the first-line imaging technique that allows the identification of the presence of a hypoechoic mass in the liver that is suspected to be ICC. CT imaging is the most useful imaging modality for the diagnosis of ICC because it shows the location of the tumor, the possible multifocality of the lesion, the presence of venous or arterial invasion, the presence of lymphadenopathy or distant metastases [53]. The typical contrast enhancement pattern with hyper-density in the late venous phase is characteristic of ICC. Other characteristics are the segmental dilation of peripheral bile ducts and retraction of Glisson's capsule in the segments near the tumor. Magnetic resonance imaging (MRI) is also important for the assessment of the extent of involvement along the bile duct and to detect the presence of satellite nodules. When contrast-enhanced methods are used, MRI allows for the detection and better definition of the presence of vascular involvement [53]. PET still has a limited role in diagnostics because of low sensitivity and specificity. However, it can be useful for the detection of distant metastases [53].

Staging Systems

The most common staging systems are the International Union Against Cancer/American Joint Committee on Cancer (UICC/AJCC) TNM classification (7th edition) [20] and the Liver Cancer Study Group of Japan (LCSGJ) TNM classification [54].

UICC/AJCC TNM Classification (7th Edition)

The UICC/AJCC TNM classification (7th edition) was published in 2010 [20] after several criticisms were raised with regard to the 6th edition. The 6th edition of UICC/AJCC TNM classification for ICC was the same for HCC due to the lack of prognostic data with respect to ICC. Nevertheless, its prognostic value has never been validated in case series of literature. In addition, ICC and HCC exhibit different neoplastic behaviors and have different prognoses. Therefore, the UICC/AJCC TNM classification 7th edition proposed a different classification for ICC. It focused on vascular invasion, the multinodularity of the tumor and the invasion into adjacent structures regardless of the size, and incorporated the pattern of growth first described in 1997 by the LCSGJ. Remarkably, the periductal infiltrating pattern was classified as T4, and regional lymph-nodal involvement was classified as N1. As in the Japanese classification, the presence of tumor in the celiac, periaortic and caval lymph-nodes is considered to be distant metastasis (M1). The prognostic value of the UICC/AJCC TNM classification 7th edition was validated by a recent multicenter analysis of 434 patients who underwent curative resection for ICC [55].

The LCSGJ TNM Classifications

This classification is used for the MF type of ICC. It evaluates three criteria: single nodule, tumor 2 cm or less and no invasion into the portal vein, hepatic vein or serous membrane. This staging system defines a solitary tumor without vascular invasion as stage I, a solitary tumor with vascular invasion as stage II, multiple tumors with or without vascular invasion as stage IIIA, a tumor with regional lymph node metastasis as stage IIIB, and a tumor with distant metastases as stage IV. In this system, tumor size is excluded from the T factor [54].

Prognostic Factors

Pattern of Growth

The macroscopic pattern of growth of the types of ICC (MF, PI, GI) reflects the different biological behaviors and the tumor spread. The MF type is the most frequent (60-70% of cases). This type is associated with an early portal invasion in 45% of cases, and satellite nodules are present in 36% of cases. Lymph node involvement is present in approximately 30% of cases. The 5-year survival rate reported in the literature varies between 25% and 48% [54, 56]. Among all cases of resected ICC, the IG type is found in 8% to 23% of cases. It presents as a papillary-like tumor, and it is well differentiated in most cases with a low frequency of lymph-nodal, vascular or perineural invasion. The long-term survival of patients with IG-ICC after surgical resection is good, with a 5-year survival of 40-80%. The survival for patients with type IG ICC is significantly longer than that for patients with the MF and PI types and is also associated with the presence of lymph-node metastases [57].

The PI type has a worse prognosis than the other two types. This form is found in 15-35% of cases and is associated with biliary, vascular and lymphatic infiltration at the hepatic hilum. The 5-year survival rate in these patients is less than 40% [58]. The mixed form MF + PI is found in 25%-45% of patients. This form has the worst prognosis because patients are typically at a more advanced stage at the time of diagnosis; they also have a higher frequency of lymph node metastases as well as vascular invasion and intrahepatic metastases. The long-term survival is poor, with less than 10% of patients alive at 5 years [57].

Local Extension

The local extent of the tumor is related to size, multifocality, vascular invasion, and invasion of the common bile duct. The size of the tumor is an important factor that determines the prognosis. Indeed, the 5-year survival in patients with a mass less than 3 cm in size is 42%, while in patients with a mass greater than 6 cm, the survival is reduced to 0% [59]. The presence of satellite nodules, in the literature, has been reported in 20-30% of patients, with a poor 5-year survival (0-7%)[59, 60]. Portal infiltration is an important negative prognostic factor for patients with ICC. Survival was significantly greater in patients without portal involvement than in those with macroscopic portal infiltration; these patients have a 3-year survival of 46% and 0%, respectively [61].

Lymph node Involvement

In the literature, the presence of lymph node metastases ranges from 7% to 73%. It is a major prognostic factor, as patients with N+ demonstrate a 5-year survival between 0% and 20% [62]. The frequency of lymph node involvement in the IG form is significantly lower than in the other forms, while the frequency of lymph node involvement in the mixed type MF + PI is significantly higher. According to some series, lymph-nodal involvement does not exceed 20% in the former, while it reaches 80% in the latter. Lymph node involvement is also related to the stage of disease, and according to some studies, it is present in 80% of patients with advanced stage disease (T4) [63]. The frequency of lymph node metastases is also related to the site of the tumor and is reported to be higher in tumors with hilar involvement than in those with peripheral growth (75 vs 45%, respectively) [64].

Macro- and Microscopic Biological Pattern

The histological aspects related to the prognosis are: cell differentiation, and lymphatic and perineural vascular invasion. With regards to cell differentiation, the well or moderately differentiated tumors have a better prognosis than those that are poorly differentiated. The 5-year survival rates are 50%, 39% and 0% for well, moderately or poorly differentiated tumors, respectively [64]. Lymphatic vessel invasion is a poor prognostic factor for survival according to the literature [65], and none of the patients with lymphatic involvement have survival rates that exceed 3 years, while a 5-year survival is reported in 70% of patients without lymphatic invasion [66]. According to some studies, patients with perineural invasion had a 5-year survival of less than 10%, while it exceeds 60% in patients without such involvement. Furthermore, perineural invasion is associated with a high frequency of lymph node metastases and the presence of vascular invasion [65]. Several biological and molecular prognostic factors have been identified in ICC. A reduced expression of IL-6 and p27kip1, and mutations in k-ras, p53, E-cadherin, α-catenin and β-catenin are associated with advanced malignancies, poor differentiation and early recurrence [67]. Unfortunately, these molecular markers still have no clinical application.

Surgical Treatment

For a correct preoperative assessment of the resectability of a tumor, several aspects must be considered: the performance status of the patient, liver function, the volume of the future remnant liver, the presence of lobe atrophy, the extension of the tumor, the vascular involvement, the lymph node involvement, and the presence of distant metastasis [68]. The resectability of tumors in patients with ICC ranges from 20%-70% according to published studies [69] and depends on the presence of intrahepatic or distant metastases, vascular invasion or peritoneal carcinomatosis. Radical surgical resection (R0) is the treatment of choice and the only one that is able to achieve long-term survival. In order to achieve radical resection, a major hepatectomy is often required. In addition, the resection of the extrahepatic bile duct, hilar vascular structures, the vena cava and the diaphragm may also be required [68, 69]. Because ICC usually arises in non-cirrhotic livers, a major hepatic resection can be performed with low morbidity and mortality. The complication rate is related to the extent of liver resection and varies between 35% in minor hepatectomies and 55% in major liver resections, but is also associated with vascular or diaphragmatic resection [60]. In most studies, the mortality is lower than 5% and is often related to major liver resections or is associated with vascular or bile duct resections. Radical surgical resection (R0) is the only factor that allows for satisfactory long-term survival and has a reported 5-year survival that can reach 40-60% in selected patients [68, 69]. The five-year survival for patients who undergo non-radical resection (R1) ranges between 0% and 25% [68].

Liver Transplantation (OLT)

Whereas excellent long-term, recurrence-free survival of patients has been achieved for hilar cholangiocarcinoma using a regimen of preoperative staging and neoadjuvant chemoradiation treatment followed by OLT [70], the role of OLT in the treatment of unresectable ICC is controversial. Despite the first instances in which poor survival (28% at 5 years) and high recurrence rates (up to 78%) were reported, recent papers in the literature have described promising results, especially when neoadjuvant and adjuvant therapies were given. Indeed, the reported survival rate in the patients who received these treatments ranges from 33% to 46% [71] in earlier series. Nevertheless, a small case series and a short follow-up cannot allow for definitive conclusions.

Chemotherapy

Numerous clinical trials have been conducted on a variety of chemotherapy regimens for the treatment of patients with ICC. Most trials had significant limitations, including lack of a control arm, small sample size, and the inclusion of a spectrum of heterogeneous tumor types. Because the response rate to single-agent 5-fluorouracil-based or gemcitabine-based systemic chemotherapy is only approximately 10% to 30% [72], currently, the most widely used therapy is based on gemcitabine and cisplatin. This approach has demonstrated an improved progression-free survival and overall survival (11.7 months vs 8.1 months) compared with gemcitabine alone [73].

Disease Recurrence

Recurrence is common even after R0 resection and arises in 40-80% of cases, and it generally occurs early (within 2 years in 86% of patients). The most frequent sites of recurrence are the liver (74%), the peritoneum (22%), lymph nodes and bone (11%) [63]. In the literature, the following factors are identified and are related to recurrence: hilar involvement, size of the tumor, portal involvement, presence of lymph node metastases, high serum levels of Ca 19-9 [63]. Another factor that is related to the onset of a high rate of recurrence is the gross macroscopic type of growth. The frequency of recurrence is significantly higher in the PI form compared to the MF form. The macroscopic type of growth also determines the site of recurrence. The MF form of ICC is particularly associated with an increased frequency of intrahepatic recurrences (68% of all recurrences), while lymph-nodal recurrence is more frequent in the MF + PI and PI forms of ICC. The treatment of recurrent tumors varies and is dependent on the location and extension of the tumor; in most cases, treatment is only palliative. In isolated cases, it is possible to reach a long-term survival after resection of an intrahepatic recurrence [74]. In very selected cases, surgical treatment including transplantation, has offered good results with regards to long-term survival [65, 75]. However, the clear indications of the proper treatment of recurrent tumors, both surgical and palliative, have not yet been clearly established in the literature.

Other Primary Liver Cancers

Fibrolamellar Hepatocellular Carcinoma

Fibrolamellar hepatocellular carcinoma (FL-HCC) is a rare variant of conventional HCC. The incidence rate has been estimated at 0.02 per 100,000 in the U.S. (approximately 100 times less common than other HCCs) [49]. It differs from HCC in most of its pathological and clinical characteristics. FL-HCC typically affects younger patients, ranging from 14 to 33 years in most series, and it constitutes one of the major primary liver tumors in younger patients. The majority of patients are not affected by underlying liver disease. In a recent review of the literature, only 3% of patients had underlying cirrhosis, while hepatitis B infection was present in 2% and hepatitis C was present in 1% [76]. The serum level of alpha-fetoprotein is elevated in approximately 10% of cases. The patients present with a few non-specific symptoms, such as fatigue or weight loss, and thus the diagnosis is almost always made by ultrasound. FL-HCC often appears as a large nodular mass, up to 20 cm in size. In contrast to HCC, FL-HCC is associated with a high rate of lymph node metastasis. The treatment that offers the best results is surgery, either aggressive liver resection or liver transplantation. Due to the high rate of lymph-node involvement at presentation, hilar lymphadenectomy should be performed. The reported 1-, 3- and 5-year overall survival ranged from 82% to 100%, 58% to 100%, and 58% to 82%, respectively, after liver resection [77] and 63% to 100%, 43% to 75%, and 29% to 55%, respectively, after liver transplantation [78]. Older age, resectability, impaired liver function, larger tumor size, multiple tumor foci, presence of comorbidities and advanced stage of disease (lymph nodal or distant metastases and vascular invasion) are factors that impaired the overall and disease-free survival. Despite the advanced stage at diagnosis, FL-HCC seems to have a fairly good prognosis, with a 5-year survival rate that is twice as high as that of HCC [79]. Nevertheless, recent data seem to show that the long-term outcome in patients with FL-HCC does not differ from that of patients with HCC when matched with patients without cirrhosis [80, 81].

Epithelioid Hemangioendothelioma

Epithelioid hemangioendothelioma (EH, Figure 4) is a primary liver cancer that originates from endothelial tissue. It has an incidence of less than one in one million. The male:female ratio is 1:2. Even if some possible etiologic factors of EH have been described, including oral contraceptives, vinyl chloride, exposure to asbestos or thorotrast, major trauma to the liver, underlying liver disease, primary biliary cirrhosis, and alcohol consumption, no clear etiological correlation has been described. Its presentation is either asymptomatic or is associated with non-specific symptoms (e.g., pain in the upper right abdominal quadrant, weight loss, anorexia) in 25% of patients [82]. The laboratoristic serum values or tumor markers are only slightly elevated or are within the normal range. Radiological findings with CT or MRI often show one or more masses in the liver with hypervascularization, but the diagnosis still poses a challenge. In almost all cases, a definitive diagnosis requires a histopathologic analysis with a biopsy. At presentation, this disease appears multifocal in 87% of cases, with an extrahepatic spread, such as to the lung, lymph nodes or peritoneum, in almost 37% of patients [82]. There is no generally accepted strategy for the treatment of HHE because of its rarity, heterogeneous status, and variable clinical outcome. The management options for patients with HHE include resection, liver transplantation, chemotherapy, and radiotherapy. Liver resection is indicated when the tumor is technically resectable, even in cases of multinodular bilobar spread. In a recent case series, liver resection demonstrated a 1-, 3- and 5-year overall survival of 100%, 86% and 86%, respectively, and a disease-free survival of 78%, 62% and 62%, respectively [83]. Liver transplantation showed good results despite the limited outcome data that are available from single-institution studies. Long-term survival data from recent reviews have demonstrated a 1-year survival rate of 80% or higher, and 5-year survival rates ranged from 54.5% to 83%[83, 84]. The experience with systemic or locoregional chemotherapy, TACE, and radiotherapy is low and generally of limited value, especially as a first-line therapy [82].

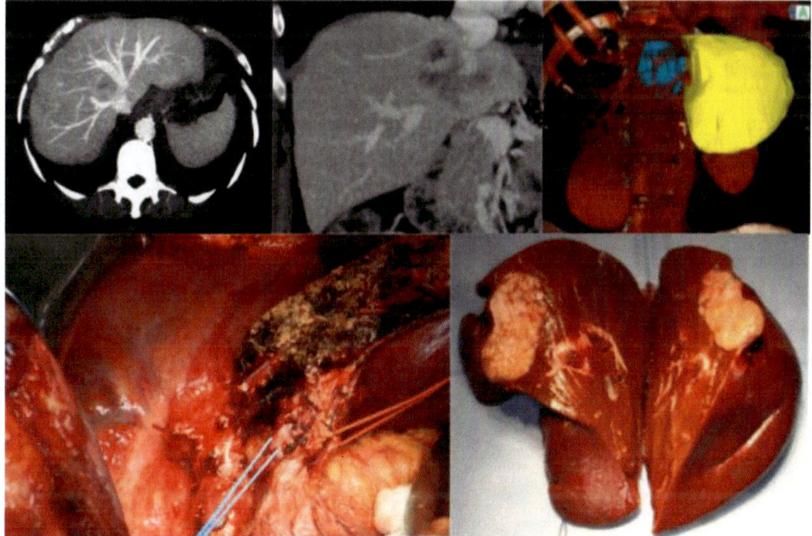

Figure 3. ICC nodules in the right lobe of the liver that surround but do not infiltrate the middle hepatic vein, as demonstrated in preoperative planning with 3-D reconstruction. Right hepatectomy was performed with negative margins.

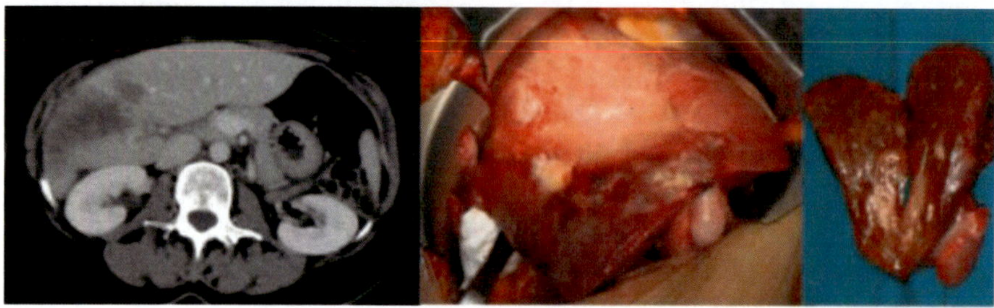

Figure 4. The onset of epithelioid hemangioendothelioma in a 19-year-old male patient. Right hepatectomy was performed with radical intent.

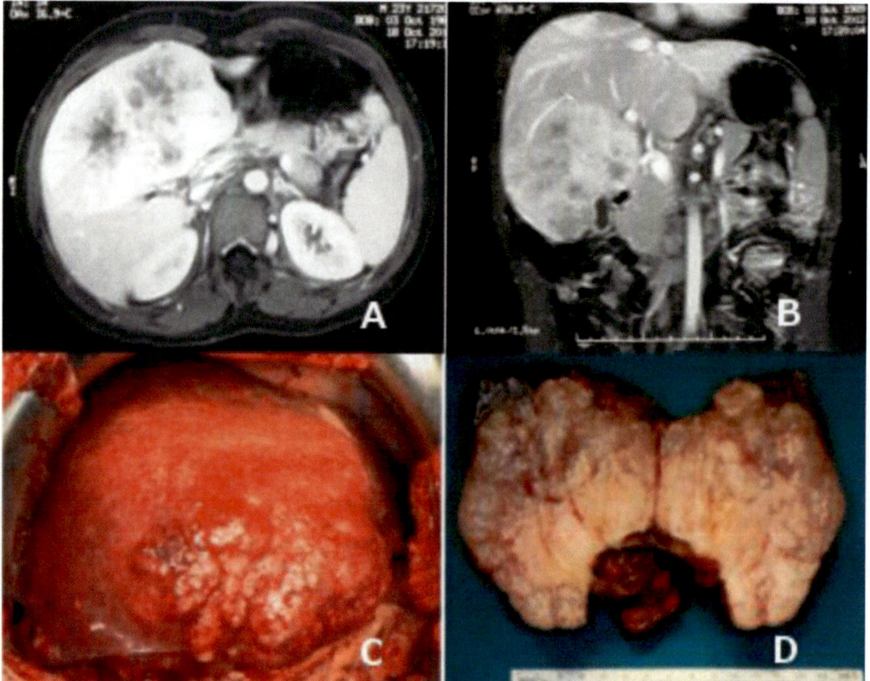

Figure 5. Hepatoblastoma in the right hepatic lobe.

Hepatoblastoma

Hepatoblastoma is the most common primary liver cancer in childhood, but it is extremely rare in adults. A recent review of studies published in English [85] reported only 40 patients who were affected by hepatoblastoma since 1958. The median age of presentation is in the fourth decade, but the majority of patients were in the second decade of life. It presents as a single, large nodule in the liver in almost 80% of cases. The symptoms and laboratory tests are non-specific, and radiological imaging has a limited valueTherefore, a biopsy-proven histological examination often leads to a definitive diagnosis. There is no standardized management of adult hepatoblastoma. Radical surgical excision appears to be the 'gold standard' for curative therapy. Chemotherapy can be used as neo- or adjuvant, and it is based on platinum, adriamycin, irinotecan and pirarubicin. The prognosis of hepatoblastoma is extremely poor. The median survival is only 4 months with a 1-year survival of 29.6%. Younger patients had significantly better prognoses than older patients [85].

Sarcoma

Primary sarcomas of the liver account for less than 1% of all hepatic malignancies. Based on the most prevalent cell type in the nodule, they are called angiosarcoma, embryonal sarcoma, leiomyosarcoma, epithelioid hemangioendothelioma, fibrosarcoma, or malignant fibrous histiocytoma. A diagnosis can be performed in patients of all ages, and often, these tumors are occasionally discovered during a routine ultrasound. Radical resection, which has a median survival of 39 months, is the treatment of choice [86].

Primary Hepatic Lymphoma

While involvement of the liver in non–Hodgkin's lymphoma is common, the occurrence of primary hepatic lymphoma is rare. Fewer than one hundred cases are described in the English language literature, and most of them are from autoptic studies. An increased incidence has been described in the past three decades, especially in immunosuppressed patients. With respect to the radiological findings, primary hepatic lymphoma often appears as a single nodule in the liver, but multiple lesions can occur, especially in patients with immunodeficiency. A definitive diagnosis can be pursued only by histological-proven biopsy. Liver resection can offer good long-term results, especially in the case of solitary nodules, while chemotherapy can prolong survival in patients with advanced disease [87].

Combined Hepatocellular and Cholangiocarcinoma

Combined hepatocellular and cholangiocarcinoma is a primary liver cancer that comprises the histological features of both HCC and ICC. It accounts for 0.4–14.2% of all primary liver carcinomas and varies greatly with geographical location. Its risk factors are a combination of those of both HCC and CCC. Its presentation can mimic HCC or ICC and depends on the most prevalent cell type. This means that it can sometimes be misdiagnosed. As with ICC, a lymph-nodal spread is observed in 30% of cases. Liver resection that includes the hilar lymph node is the treatment of choice. The reported median survival ranges from 20 to 47 months. Vascular and lymph node invasion and the presence of satellite metastases have been suggested to be significant predictors of poor outcome after resection. The recurrence rate is high and is approximately 95% within 2 years after resection, which accounts for the poor prognosis [88].

References

[1] Ferlay, J., D.M. Parkin, and E. Steliarova-Foucher, Estimates of cancer incidence and mortality in Europe in 2008. *Eur J Cancer,* 2010. *46*(4): p. 765-81.

[2] Srivatanakul, P., H. Sriplung, and S. Deerasamee, Epidemiology of liver cancer: an overview. *Asian Pac J Cancer Prev,* 2004. *5*(2): p. 118-25.

[3] Tsukuma, H., et al., Liver cancer and its prevention. *Asian Pac J Cancer Prev*, 2005. *6*(3): p. 244-50.

[4] Jemal, A., et al., Global cancer statistics. *CA Cancer J Clin,* 2011. *61*(2): p. 69-90.

[5] Bruix, J. and M. Sherman, Management of hepatocellular carcinoma. *Hepatology,* 2005. *42*(5): p. 1208-36.

[6] Bosetti, C., et al., Trends in mortality from hepatocellular carcinoma in Europe, 1980-2004. *Hepatology,* 2008. *48*(1): p. 137-45.

[7] Ioannou, G.N., et al., The prevalence of cirrhosis and hepatocellular carcinoma in patients with human immunodeficiency virus infection. *Hepatology*, 2013. *57*(1): p. 249-57.

[8] Kadayifci, A., et al., Clinical and pathologic risk factors for atherosclerosis in cirrhosis: a comparison between NASH-related cirrhosis and cirrhosis due to other aetiologies. *J Hepatol,* 2008. *49*(4): p. 595-9.

[9] Bruix, J., et al., Clinical decision making and research in hepatocellular carcinoma: pivotal role of imaging techniques. *Hepatology,* 2011. *54*(6): p. 2238-44.

[10] Kudo, M., et al., Management of hepatocellular carcinoma in Japan: Consensus-Based Clinical Practice Guidelines proposed by the Japan Society of Hepatology (JSH) 2010 updated version. *Dig Dis,* 2011. *29*(3): p. 339-64.

[11] EASL-EORTC clinical practice guidelines: management of hepatocellular carcinoma. *J Hepatol,* 2012. *56*(4): p. 908-43.

[12] Cillo, U., et al., The critical issue of hepatocellular carcinoma prognostic classification: which is the best tool available? *J Hepatol,* 2004. *40*(1): p. 124-31.

[13] Guglielmi, A., et al., Comparison of seven staging systems in cirrhotic patients with hepatocellular carcinoma in a cohort of patients who underwent radiofrequency ablation with complete response. *Am J Gastroenterol,* 2008. *103*(3): p. 597-604.

[14] Grieco, A., et al., Prognostic factors for survival in patients with early-intermediate hepatocellular carcinoma undergoing non-surgical therapy: comparison of Okuda, CLIP, and BCLC staging systems in a single Italian centre. *Gut,* 2005. *54*(3): p. 411-8.

[15] Marrero, J.A., et al., Prognosis of hepatocellular carcinoma: comparison of 7 staging systems in an American cohort. *Hepatology,* 2005. *41*(4): p. 707-16.

[16] Sala, M., et al., Prognostic prediction in patients with hepatocellular carcinoma. *Semin Liver Dis,* 2005. *25*(2): p. 171-80.

[17] Ruzzenente, A., et al., Hepatocellular carcinoma in cirrhotic patients with portal hypertension: is liver resection always contraindicated? *World J Gastroenterol,* 2011. *17*(46): p. 5083-8.

[18] Chang, W.T., et al., Hepatic resection can provide long-term survival of patients with non-early-stage hepatocellular carcinoma: extending the indication for resection? *Surgery,* 2012. *152*(5): p. 809-20.

[19] Ruzzenente, A., et al., Is liver resection justified in advanced hepatocellular carcinoma? Results of an observational study in 464 patients. *J Gastrointest Surg, 2009. 13*(7): p. 1313-20.

[20] Sobin, L.H. and C.C. Compton, TNM seventh edition: what's new, what's changed: communication from the International Union Against Cancer and the American Joint Committee on Cancer. *Cancer,* 2010. *116*(22): p. 5336-9.

[21] A new prognostic system for hepatocellular carcinoma: a retrospective study of 435 patients: the Cancer of the Liver Italian Program (CLIP) investigators. *Hepatology,* 1998. *28*(3): p. 751-5.

[22] Ueno, S., et al., Discrimination value of the new western prognostic system (CLIP score) for hepatocellular carcinoma in 662 Japanese patients. Cancer of the Liver Italian Program. *Hepatology,* 2001. *34*(3): p. 529-34.

[23] Levy, I. and M. Sherman, Staging of hepatocellular carcinoma: assessment of the CLIP, Okuda, and Child-Pugh staging systems in a cohort of 257 patients in Toronto. *Gut,* 2002. *50*(6): p. 881-5.

[24] Kudo, M., H. Chung, and Y. Osaki, Prognostic staging system for hepatocellular carcinoma (CLIP score): its value and limitations, and a proposal for a new staging system, the Japan Integrated Staging Score (JIS score). *J Gastroenterol,* 2003. *38*(3): p. 207-15.

[25] Llovet, J.M. and J. Bruix, Systematic review of randomized trials for unresectable hepatocellular carcinoma: Chemoembolization improves survival. *Hepatology,* 2003. *37*(2): p. 429-42.

[26] Mazzaferro, V., et al., Liver transplantation for hepatocellular carcinoma. *Ann Surg Oncol,* 2008. *15*(4): p. 1001-7.

[27] Guglielmi, A., et al., How much remnant is enough in liver resection? *Dig Surg,* 2012. *29*(1): p. 6-17.

[28] Guglielmi, A., et al., Radiofrequency ablation versus surgical resection for the treatment of hepatocellular carcinoma in cirrhosis. *J Gastrointest Surg,* 2008. *12*(1): p. 192-8.

[29] Ruzzenente, A., et al., Surgical resection versus local ablation for HCC on cirrhosis: results from a propensity case-matched study. *J Gastrointest Surg,* 2012. *16*(2): p. 301-11; discussion 311.

[30] Cucchetti, A., et al., Systematic review of surgical resection vs radiofrequency ablation for hepatocellular carcinoma. *World J Gastroenterol,* 2013. *19*(26): p. 4106-18.

[31] EASL-EORTC clinical practice guidelines: management of hepatocellular carcinoma. Eur J Cancer, 2012. *48*(5): p. 599-641.

[32] Lencioni, R., et al., Treatment of intermediate/advanced hepatocellular carcinoma in the clinic: how can outcomes be improved? *Oncologist,* 2010. *15 Suppl 4*: p. 42-52.

[33] Piscaglia, F. and L. Bolondi, The intermediate hepatocellular carcinoma stage: Should treatment be expanded? *Dig Liver Dis,* 2010. *42 Suppl 3*: p. S258-63.

[34] Yuen, M.F., et al., Transarterial chemoembolization for inoperable, early stage hepatocellular carcinoma in patients with Child-Pugh grade A and B: results of a comparative study in 96 Chinese patients. *Am J Gastroenterol,* 2003. *98*(5): p. 1181-5.

[35] Zhang, Z.M., et al., Therapeutic options for intermediate-advanced hepatocellular carcinoma. *World J Gastroenterol,* 2011. *17*(13): p. 1685-9.

[36] Lopez, R.R., Jr., et al., Comparison of transarterial chemoembolization in patients with unresectable, diffuse vs focal hepatocellular carcinoma. *Arch Surg,* 2002. *137*(6): p. 653-7; discussion 657-8.

[37] Dufour, J.F., et al., Intermediate hepatocellular carcinoma: current treatments and future perspectives. *Ann Oncol,* 2013. *24 Suppl 2*: p. ii24-9.

[38] Sangro, B., M. Inarrairaegui, and J.I. Bilbao, Radioembolization for hepatocellular carcinoma. *J Hepatol,* 2012. *56*(2): p. 464-73.

[39] Llovet, J.M., et al., Sorafenib in advanced hepatocellular carcinoma. *N Engl J Med,* 2008. *359*(4): p. 378-90.

[40] Cheng, A.L., et al., Efficacy and safety of sorafenib in patients in the Asia-Pacific region with advanced hepatocellular carcinoma: a phase III randomised, double-blind, placebo-controlled trial. *Lancet Oncol,* 2009. *10*(1): p. 25-34.

[41] Kaneko, S., et al., Guideline on the use of new anticancer drugs for the treatment of Hepatocellular Carcinoma 2010 update. *Hepatol Res,* 2012. *42*(6): p. 523-42.

[42] Shah, S.A., et al., Recurrence after liver resection for hepatocellular carcinoma: risk factors, treatment, and outcomes. *Surgery,* 2007. *141*(3): p. 330-9.

[43] Nagao, T., et al., Postoperative recurrence of hepatocellular carcinoma. *Ann Surg,* 1990. *211*(1): p. 28-33.

[44] Shah, S.A., et al., An analysis of resection vs transplantation for early hepatocellular carcinoma: defining the optimal therapy at a single institution. *Ann Surg Oncol,* 2007. *14*(9): p. 2608-14.

[45] Pedica, F., et al., A re-emerging marker for prognosis in hepatocellular carcinoma: the add-value of fishing c-myc gene for early relapse. *PLoS One,* 2013. *8*(7): p. e68203.

[46] Ehrenfried, J.A. and J.N. Vauthey, Biliary tract cancer. *Curr Opin Gastroenterol,* 1999. *15*(5): p. 430-5.

[47] Patel, T., Cholangiocarcinoma. *Nat Clin Pract Gastroenterol Hepatol, 2006. 3*(1): p. 33-42.

[48] Khan, S.A., et al., Guidelines for the diagnosis and treatment of cholangiocarcinoma: consensus document. *Gut,* 2002. *51 Suppl 6*: p. VI1-9.

[49] Shaib, Y. and H.B. El-Serag, The epidemiology of cholangiocarcinoma. *Semin Liver Dis,* 2004. *24*(2): p. 115-25.

[50] Shaib, Y.H., et al., Rising incidence of intrahepatic cholangiocarcinoma in the United States: a true increase? *J Hepatol,* 2004. *40*(3): p. 472-7.

[51] J, T., *Classification of primary liver cancer.*2004.

[52] Patel, A.H., et al., The utility of CA 19-9 in the diagnoses of cholangiocarcinoma in patients without primary sclerosing cholangitis. *Am J Gastroenterol,* 2000. *95*(1): p. 204-7.

[53] Zhang, Y., et al., Intrahepatic peripheral cholangiocarcinoma: comparison of dynamic CT and dynamic MRI. J Comput Assist Tomogr, 1999. *23*(5): p. 670-7.

[54] Yamasaki, S., Intrahepatic cholangiocarcinoma: macroscopic type and stage classification. *J Hepatobiliary Pancreat Surg,* 2003. *10*(4): p. 288-91.

[55] Ribero, D., et al., Comparison of the prognostic accuracy of the sixth and seventh editions of the TNM classification for intrahepatic cholangiocarcinoma. *HPB* (Oxford), 2011. *13*(3): p. 198-205.

[56] Ikai, I., et al., Report of the 16th follow-up survey of primary liver cancer. Hepatol Res, 2005. *32*(3): p. 163-72.

[57] Yeh, C.N., et al., Hepatic resection of the intraductal papillary type of peripheral cholangiocarcinoma. *Ann Surg Oncol,* 2004. *11*(6): p. 606-11.

[58] Morimoto, Y., et al., Long-term survival and prognostic factors in the surgical treatment for intrahepatic cholangiocarcinoma. *J Hepatobiliary Pancreat Surg,* 2003. *10*(6): p. 432-40.

[59] Isa, T., et al., Predictive factors for long-term survival in patients with intrahepatic cholangiocarcinoma. *Am J Surg,* 2001. *181*(6): p. 507-11.

[60] Suzuki, S., et al., Clinicopathological prognostic factors and impact of surgical treatment of mass-forming intrahepatic cholangiocarcinoma. *World J Surg,* 2002. *26*(6): p. 687-93.

[61] Okabayashi, T., et al., A new staging system for mass-forming intrahepatic cholangiocarcinoma: analysis of preoperative and postoperative variables. *Cancer,* 2001. *92*(9): p. 2374-83.

[62] Nakagawa, T., et al., Number of lymph node metastases is a significant prognostic factor in intrahepatic cholangiocarcinoma. *World J Surg,* 2005. *29*(6): p. 728-33.

[63] Miwa, S., et al., Predictive factors for intrahepatic cholangiocarcinoma recurrence in the liver following surgery. *J Gastroenterol,* 2006. *41*(9): p. 893-900.
[64] Isaji, S., et al., Clinicopathological features and outcome of hepatic resection for intrahepatic cholangiocarcinoma in Japan. *J Hepatobiliary Pancreat Surg,* 1999. *6*(2): p. 108-16.
[65] Nakagohri, T., et al., Aggressive surgical resection for hilar-invasive and peripheral intrahepatic cholangiocarcinoma. *World J Surg,* 2003. *27*(3): p. 289-93.
[66] Uenishi, T., et al., Histologic factors affecting prognosis following hepatectomy for intrahepatic cholangiocarcinoma. *World J Surg, 2001. 25(7): p. 865-9.*
[67] Nakanuma, Y., et al., Anatomic and molecular pathology of intrahepatic cholangiocarcinoma. *J Hepatobiliary Pancreat Surg,* 2003. *10*(4): p. 265-81.
[68] Guglielmi, A., et al., Intrahepatic cholangiocarcinoma: prognostic factors after surgical resection. *World J Surg,* 2009. *33*(6): p. 1247-54.
[69] Lang, H., et al., Extended hepatectomy for intrahepatic cholangiocellular carcinoma (ICC): when is it worthwhile? Single center experience with 27 resections in 50 patients over a 5-year period. *Ann Surg,* 2005. *241*(1): p. 134-43.
[70] Rea, D.J., et al., Liver transplantation with neoadjuvant chemoradiation is more effective than resection for hilar cholangiocarcinoma. *Ann Surg, 2005. 242*(3): p. 451-8; discussion 458-61.
[71] Hong, J.C., et al., Comparative analysis of resection and liver transplantation for intrahepatic and hilar cholangiocarcinoma: a 24-year experience in a single center. *Arch Surg,* 2011. *146*(6): p. 683-9.
[72] Kim, M.J., et al., Gemcitabine-based versus fluoropyrimidine-based chemotherapy with or without platinum in unresectable biliary tract cancer: a retrospective study. *BMC Cancer,* 2008. *8*: p. 374.
[73] Valle, J., et al., Cisplatin plus gemcitabine versus gemcitabine for biliary tract cancer. *N Engl J Med,* 2010. *362*(14): p. 1273-81.
[74] Sano, T., et al., One hundred two consecutive hepatobiliary resections for perihilar cholangiocarcinoma with zero mortality. *Ann Surg,* 2006. *244*(2): p. 240-7.
[75] Cherqui, D., et al., Intrahepatic cholangiocarcinoma. Results of aggressive surgical management. *Arch Surg,* 1995. *130*(10): p. 1073-8.

[76] Mavros, M.N., et al., A systematic review: treatment and prognosis of patients with fibrolamellar hepatocellular carcinoma. *J Am Coll Surg,* 2012. *215*(6): p. 820-30.

[77] Stipa, F., et al., Outcome of patients with fibrolamellar hepatocellular carcinoma. *Cancer,* 2006. *106*(6): p. 1331-8.

[78] El-Gazzaz, G., et al., Outcome of liver resection and transplantation for fibrolamellar hepatocellular carcinoma. *Transpl Int,* 2000. *13 Suppl 1*: p. S406-9.

[79] El-Serag, H.B. and J.A. Davila, Is fibrolamellar carcinoma different from hepatocellular carcinoma? A US population-based study. *Hepatology,* 2004. *39*(3): p. 798-803.

[80] Kakar, S., et al., Clinicopathologic features and survival in fibrolamellar carcinoma: comparison with conventional hepatocellular carcinoma with and without cirrhosis. *Mod Pathol,* 2005. *18*(11): p. 1417-23.

[81] Weeda, V.B., et al., Fibrolamellar variant of hepatocellular carcinoma does not have a better survival than conventional hepatocellular carcinoma--results and treatment recommendations from the Childhood Liver Tumour Strategy Group (SIOPEL) experience. *Eur J Cancer,* 2013. *49*(12): p. 2698-704.

[82] Mehrabi, A., et al., Primary malignant hepatic epithelioid hemangioendothelioma: a comprehensive review of the literature with emphasis on the surgical therapy. *Cancer,* 2006. *107*(9): p. 2108-21.

[83] Grotz, T.E., et al., Hepatic epithelioid haemangioendothelioma: is transplantation the only treatment option? *HPB* (Oxford), 2010. *12*(8): p. 546-53.

[84] Agrawal, N., et al., Liver transplantation in the management of hepatic epithelioid hemangioendothelioma: a single-center experience and review of the literature. *Transplant Proc,* 2011. *43*(7): p. 2647-50.

[85] Wang, Y.X. and H. Liu, Adult hepatoblastoma: systemic review of the English literature. *Dig Surg,* 2012. *29*(4): p. 323-30.

[86] Weitz, J., et al., Management of primary liver sarcomas. *Cancer,* 2007. *109*(7): p. 1391-6.

[87] Schweiger, F., R. Shinder, and S. Rubin, Primary lymphoma of the liver: a case report and review. *Can J Gastroenterol,* 2000. *14*(11): p. 955-7.

[88] Kassahun, W.T. and J. Hauss, Management of combined hepatocellular and cholangiocarcinoma. *Int J Clin Pract,* 2008. *62*(8): p. 1271-8.

In: Prognostic and Predictive Response ... ISBN: 978-1-63463-545-5
Editors: V. Canzonieri and M. Berretta

Chapter 5

Lung Cancer

Alessandra Bearz[1*], Vittore Pagan[2] and Tiziana Perin[3]

[1]Department of Medical Oncology, Centro di Riferimento Oncologico di Aviano National Cancer Institute - IRCCS Via Franco Gallini, Aviano (PN) Italy

[2]Department fo Surgical Oncology, Centro di Riferimento Oncologico di Aviano National National Cancer Institute - IRCCS Via Franco Gallini, Aviano (PN) Italy

[3]Division of Pathology Centro di Riferimento Oncologico di Aviano National National Cancer Institute - IRCCS Via Franco Gallini, Aviano (PN) Italy

Abstract

In recent years, many advances have been achieved in the field of lung cancer treatment, including the development of novel therapeutic pathways due to the knowledge of the oncologic drivers involved in the carcinogenesis of the lung as well as the involvement of new radiotherapeutic and surgical techniques. Herein we try to summarize the main guidelines for the prognostication of lung cancer and illustrate the clinical application of clinical biomarkers with predictive value.

* Corresponding author: Alessandra Bearz, Department of Medical Oncology, Centro di Riferimento Oncologico di Aviano National Cancer Institute - IRCCS Via Franco Gallini, 2 33081 Aviano (PN) Italy tel +390434659294 abearz@cro.it

Introduction

The prognosis indicates, roughly, the possibility of curing a disease and a prediction of life expectancy. The prognosis is one of patients' primary requests and is triggered immediately after the communication of a diagnosis of oncological disease. At the dawn of oncology, the prognosis was based on subjective aspects detected by the oncologists, which were later organized in a more scientific and reproducible system, through the creation of a rating scale known as the performance status score (Performance Status, PS). Subsequently, great emphasis was given to staging, with huge efforts undertaken to make staging consistent with the risk classes, reviewing the surgical series, in order to segregate patients into homogeneous classes of risk. This was based on the belief that the extension and geographical localization of the tumor was consistent with differing aggressiveness and biological disease correlating with the prediction of life expectancy. Our understanding of the importance of many other different tumor characteristics, such as histology and genetics, has changed the prognostic value of the simple anatomical features and changed the TNM prognostic importance. Although TNM is the basis to define the extent of the disease internationally, it has lost some of its prognostic importance, which now rests on many aspects of both the host and the tumor.

Clinical Prognostic Factors

Clinical features of patients with Non-Small-Cell Lung Cancer (NSCLC) at diagnosis offer some information to estimate their prognoses. Clinical features may have different importance according to different stages or settings.

Generally speaking, for every patient affected by NSCLC, PS and co-morbidity have been demonstrated to have prognostic influence on mortality. The term "co-morbidity" refers to non-cancer-related physical or mental disorders that may also affect a patient's treatment tolerance and outcome [1].

A diagnosis of adenocarcinoma, a small tumor, the absence of hoarseness, and resectability are independent factors related to good overall survival in stages I and II. Weight loss and clinical signs of SVCS are related to poor prognosis in stage III [2].

Performance Status, diagnosis of adenocarcinoma, an absence of weight loss and dyspnea, N0 or N1 disease and the ability to receive systemic therapy are good prognostic factors in stage IV. The ability to receive systemic therapy also includes parameters such as age and co-morbidities, which could affect the ability to receive systemic treatments. When patients with advanced or metastatic disease have already received a first-line treatment, their responses to first-line chemotherapy and time to progression affect the potential response after a second-line therapy. Sites of metastasis also affect prognosis. The reported incidence of brain metastases in patients with NSCLC ranges from 20% to 40% depending on whether autopsy, surgical or radiological data are reviewed. Multiple cerebral lesions are associated with poor prognosis, and median overall survival from the time of diagnosis is 4 months [3]. In a recently published survey, almost a thousand of Japanese patients [4] concerning prognostic factors and the significance of treatment after recurrence in completely resected stage I non-small cell lung cancer, the presence of metastasis at the bone and liver were prognostic factors significantly associated with a better survival rate.

In the last few years, the prognostic importance of several genetic mutations has been outlined. Epidermal growth factor receptor (EGFR) status impacts both progression free survival (PFS) and overall survival (OS); the impact of PFS is due to the outstanding response to the EGFR-inhibitor tyrosine kinase (TKI), and the impact of OS is due to the impact of EGFR TKI's on PFS and the availability of at least one more treatment in the patient's therapeutic pathway. KRAS status only negatively impacts OS [5].

EML4-ALK translocation is likely to bring about the same results observed for EGFR inhibitors, with a longer PFS with ALK inhibitors and longer OS.

For this reason, the regional diffusion and the extension of NSCLC have lost some of their importance, because it may be very different to have a NSCLC IV stage with EGFR sensitizing mutation for TKIs or without, and the same might be true for EML4-ALK as well. In this way, the genetic features should be strictly linked with classical TNM stages, as already suggested [6].

Interestingly, among clinical prognosticators, some surgery-dependent factors deserve separate description:

The "surgical" prognostic factors included here refer to NSCLC primary lung tumors; radiological, PET, and bronchoscopic prognostic factors are excluded. They are defined as predictive indicators of expected long-term post-surgical survival according to the commonly accepted clinical experiences and updated qualified sources (PUBMED search "lung cancer surgery prognosis" 2008-2013).

Prognostically adverse symptoms/signs, as indicating or proving potential local/regional invasion, may include: severe or persisting hemoptysis; pleural/pulmonary septic infection; persisting thoracic or vertebral pain; recurrent or phrenic nerve palsy; voice strength quickly fading down while speaking; respiratory wheezing; hypoxia; palpable cervical/supraclavear/ axillary lymph-nodes; retrosternal sense of oppression; venous mediastinal-syndrome; Bernard-Horner syndrome; anhidrosis of upper arm and/or hemitruncal skin; new-onset arrhythmia; and signs of pericardial involvement.

Preoperative predictive factors include unfavorable symptoms/signs as potential indicators of advanced or diffuse or aggressive disease, such as paraneoplastic syndrome, weight loss, asthenia, anorexia, or anemia; laboratory blood tests that show evidence of anemia, low albumin, high platelet count, high fibrinogen, high d-dimer, low ferritin, or low lymphocytes count; and clinical signs of metastatic spread in distant organs.

As general oncological factors, the following factors have been variably shown to be associated with poorer prognosis: male sex; age younger than 40 years; African-American ethnicity; non-adenocarcinoma histotype (vs. adenocarcinoma type, particularly GGO); nodular vs. elliptic adenocarcinomas; non- or poorly differentiated tumors; clinical stages higher than I-II and size of more than 1 cm in the T1 subset; diagnosis of lung cancer rising from clinical symptoms or signs (as opposed to a symptomatic incidental or tumors diagnosed via screenings, more often in the initial stages); short doubling time; multiple synchronous or metachronous primary lung tumors; tumors resistant to or showing minor partial response to inductive treatments (as opposed to complete or major partial response); and history of previous solid extrapulmonary malignancy.

Intraoperative Prognostic Factors

Reported unfavorable intraoperative prognostic factors related to the surgical procedure include non-radical macroscopic or microscopic resection (R1, R2); incomplete inspection and palpation of spared lung parenchyma; improper manipulation of the lung and excessively traumatic surgical maneuvers; intraoperative blood transfusion; long operation time; extrapulmonary extension of resection; and pneumonectomy.

Reported adverse intraoperative oncological-surgical prognostic factors include tumors infiltrating the visceral pleura; tumors freezing the pulmonary hilum; incisional (vs. excisional) intraoperative biopsies of neoplastic tissue; a delay of more than three months between the diagnosis and surgery; omitted or inadequate preoperative mapping of the tracheal-bronchial mucosa by bronchoscopy fluorescence when facing tumors with superficial spreading; missed or incomplete (with regard to recommended level/station and minimum number of nodes, i.e. at least 6) or non-systematic (either radical or sampling) lymphadenectomy; multiple lymph nodes per station/level (vs. a single node); mediastinal lymphadenopathy, even if single, diagnosed preoperatively (as opposed to node metastases diagnosed only after surgery); simultaneous hilar and mediastinal pathological lymph nodes; bulky hilar adenopathy (as a potential herald of occult mediastinal disease); and extracapsular spread of lymph node disease (i.e. N disease turning into T disease).

Non-Oncological Surgical Prognostic Factors

These factors deal with intra- and post-operative complications, which may decrease the overall chance of survival and eventually have a negative effect on the final prognostic outcome.

Individual negative prognosticators include an active smoking habit; any associated disease affecting the process of immunologic competence, nutrition, metabolism, tissue re-generation, or hemostasis; respiratory, cardiac, renal, hepatic, or vascular insufficiency; any concomitant active or inactive homolateral pathological disorder altering the anatomical planes so that the surgical dissection can be difficult and dangerous, such as dense and extended adhesions encasing pleura, lung, hilar structures, or lymph nodes (i.e. tuberculosis, fibrosis, silicosis, previous radiotherapy or trauma or thoracotomy); any tumor associated with pathogenic bacterial contamination of the tracheal-bronchial tree or with the pleural and pulmonary septic process, such as pneumonia, abscess, emphysema, bronchiectasis; pulmonary hypertension or arterial atheromatosis causing troublesome fragility of the pulmonary vessels to be isolated and ligated; and an impaired scarring process of the bronchial wall due to compromised vascularization or marked calcification.

Prognostic Factors Related to Surgeon/Hospital

Unfavorable factors related to surgeon/hospital, because of the potential source of increased surgical risk eventually affecting the final outcome, include an operation performed by a general surgeon (vs. a thoracic surgeon); a limited volume of thoracotomies per surgeon; a limited volume of thoracotomies per hospital; hospital lacking or only partially equipped with the modern resources necessary for the prompt diagnosis and treatment of possible complications (i.e. intensive therapy unit, thoracic endoscopy, interventional radiology and cardiology, microbiology lab, blood bank, and respiratory-physical-therapy); a lack of instrumentation or experience with advanced pathological diagnostic work-ups; and a hospital system unfit to deliver postoperative medical oncology and radiotherapy treatment.

Pathological Prognostic Factors

Pathological assessment of lung cancer is a crucial component for the diagnosis, management and prognosis of lung cancer. The International Association for the Study of Lung Cancer (IASLC) has collected data over time that form the basis of the currently used staging classification. The most relevant prognostic factors of the staging system are tumor size; presence of regional lymph node metastases, subdivided into pulmonary (N1), ipsilateral mediastinal (N2) or controlateral/supraclavicular (N3); and metastases in pleural fluid (M1a) or elsewhere (M1b). Slight adaptations have made for pleural invasion; the integrity of the elastic lamina can modify the stage. More than 100 other lung cancer prognostic markers have been published. As in other tumors, in lung cancer, predictive factors are the main determinants on which therapy decisions are based. Recently, it has become clinically relevant to distinguish between adenocarcinoma (AdC) and squamous cell carcinoma (SqCC), as this distinction is predictive for chemotherapy response, and now the chemotherapy therapy regimen differs for these histological types.

By definition, the WHO pathological classification of lung cancer is based on resection specimens (Figure 1 and Figure 2). Recently, in a collaborative effort by IASLC, the American Thoracic Society, and the European Respiratory Society, a refinement of the WHO classification has been established for AdCs, including guidelines for tumor typing on biopsies. The latter is important, as in biopsy and cytology specimens of lung cancer, the chance of sampling areas of special differentiation is considerably lower than identifying this in a resection specimen.

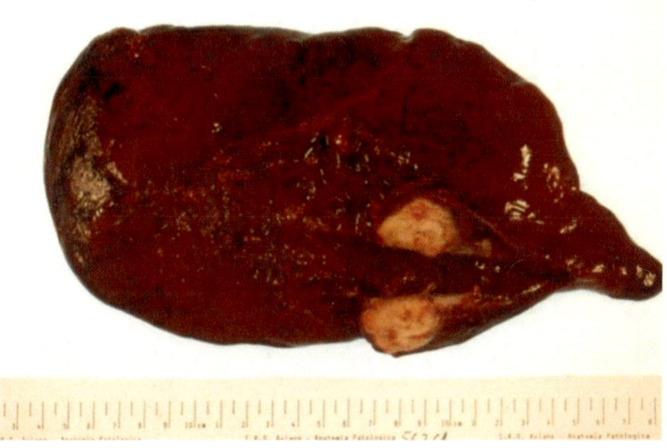

Figure 1. Surgically resected specimen containing an organ confined lung cancer.

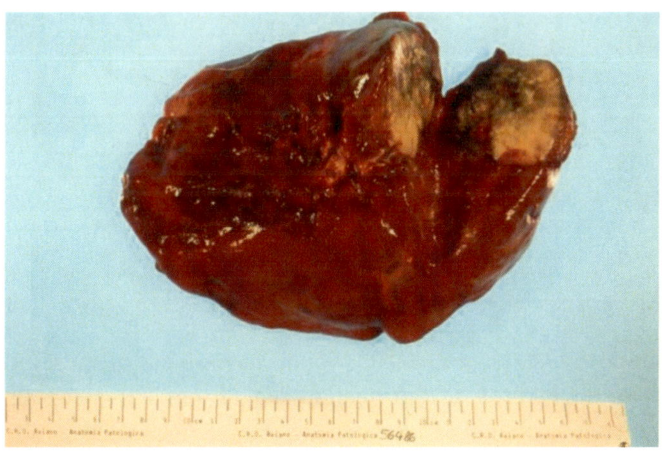

Figure 2. Lung cancer with macroscopic pleural involvement

An associated issue concerns the reliability of the diagnostic performance in distinguishing AdC from SqCC on hematoxylin- and eosin- (H&E) stained tissue sections of small biopsy samples (Figure 3). In about 35-40% of biopsies, a distinction between AdC and SqCC cannot be made. In these cases, it should be convenient to apply a panel of immunohistochemical (IHC) markers, thyroid transcription factor-1 (TTF-1), and cytokeratin 7 (CK7) to identify an adenocarcinoma component and CK5/6 and p63/p40 to identify a squamous cell carcinoma component. This simple molecular classification is extremely useful and can reduce the reporting rates of non-small-cell lung cancer, not otherwise specified (NSCLC-NOS) to less than 10%, a level that cannot be further improved. In a small fraction of tumors, both lineage-determining markers may be positive, and these tumors probably represent adenosquamous carcinoma or peripheral AdCs with squamous differentiation. Thus, this approach to lung cancer diagnosis provides biological correlations as well as predictive relevance for chemotherapy.

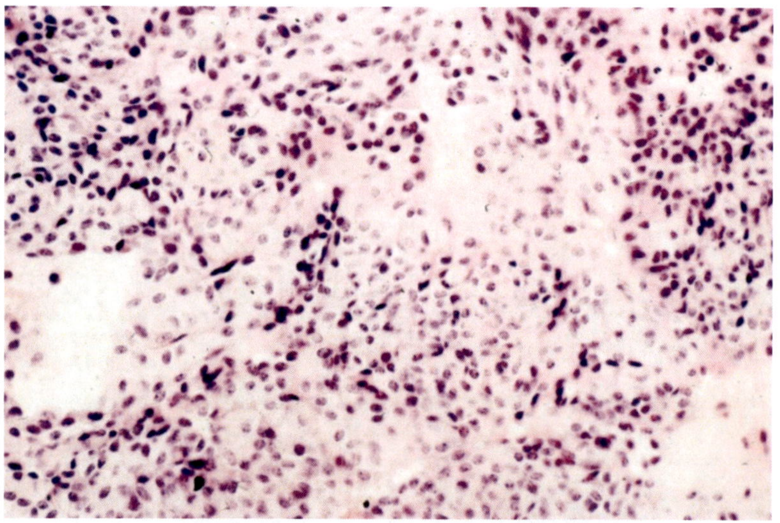

Figure 3. Lung carcinoma: diagnostic diofficulties in distinguishing AdC from SqCC on hematoxylin and eosin (H&E)-stained tissue sections.

In addition to histology and IHC typing, assessment of the expression of specific genes might provide information that is predictive for response to specific treatments; some examples include thymidylate synthase (TS), genes involved in the DNA repair of cytotoxic drug-induced damage in tumor cells, such as excision repair cross-complementation group 1 (ERCC1) and ribonucleoside-diphosphate reductase large submit (RRM1). These biomarkers are currently not in use in daily practice and need to be validated in terms of their prognostic role and the best method for their determination.

More importantly, epidermal growth factor receptor (EGFR) and anaplastic lymphoma kinase (ALK) are biomarkers currently used in clinical treatment as predictors of benefit from target therapy. Other driver biomarkers in lung cancer (point mutations, overexpression and rearrangements in specific genes including HER2, BRAF, NUT, MET, ROS1, FGFR1, KRAS, MET and PTEN) might potentially provide additional information for clinical decision making. Epidermal growth factor receptor (EGFR) and anaplastic lymphoma kinase (ALK) should be tested in all patients with advanced adenocarcinoma of the lung.

EGFR

EGFR mutation analysis is the best predictive marker for the use of EGFR-TKI therapy in NSCLC. Deletions in exon 19 and L8558R point mutation in exon 21 occur most frequently and are associated with a response rate of approximately 70% to EGFR-TKI therapy.

In daily histopathological practice, it is important to be aware of the analytical sensitivity (the minimum percentage of tumor cells in the analyzed cell sample required for a positive test result) of the EGFR mutation test. When Sanger sequencing is used, this is generally around 30-50% while more sensitive sequencing techniques reach a sensitivity of 1-10%. In particular, in bronchial biopsies, low numbers of tumor cells may be present, which is incompatible with a positive result in Sanger sequencing, but also, potentially, in next-generation sequencing. The analytical sensitivity of next-generation sequencing in clinical application currently varies between 1-10%, depending on the number of reads performed(100-5000).

The required amount of input DNA varies between 10-150 ng, which is difficult to obtain on bronchial biopsies. A possible alternative analytical technique is the use of EGFR mutation-specific antibodies in IHC, which identify a 15bp detection in exon 19 and an L858R point mutation in exon 21. Currently, these are not recommended for predictive testing, as the detection sensitivity, in particular for less frequent exon 19 deletions, is moderate, the 15bp deletion being better recognized than the 18 or 12 bp deletions. However, when a limited number of cells is available, such as in a cytological sample, the application of IHC with these mutation-specific antibodies may be useful.

ALK

In NSCLC cells, a small inversion within chromosome 2p results in a fusion gene comprising portions of the EML4 and ALK genes. ALK-positive cases have been detected in all histological subtypes of AdC, but a preference for a solid signet-ring cell pattern and a mucinous cribriform pattern with a lack of significant nuclear pleomorphism seems to exist. To establish ALK-positive status, any validated test (IHC ,FISH or RT-PCR) can be used.

HER2

HER2 is a member of the HER (EGFR) family of tyrosine kinase receptors, with no specific ligand, and when activated, is able to form dimers with other EGFR family members. HER2 is expressed in about 24% of NSCLC. In a meta-analysis of 40 published studies, HER2 IHC overexpression was associated with poor prognosis in AdCs. HER2 amplification determined by FISH was not prognostic. Whether amplification is associated with response to therapy is not clear.

BRAF

RAF proteins are serine/threonine kinase downstream of RAS in the RAS-RAF-ERK-MAPK pathway. Among them, the BRAF gene is most frequently mutated in NSCLC (1-3% of AdCs). (In contrast to melanoma, about 50% of the mutations are non-V600E mutations). BRAF mutations are responsible for permanent activation of downstream MAPK2, and 3 are mutually exclusive with EGFR and RAS mutations. In contrast to other driver mutations, BRAF mutations occur more frequently in smokers than in non-smokers.

RET

RET (rearranged during transfection) is a proto-oncogene on chromosome 10 encoding a receptor tyrosine kinase growth factor of the glial-derived neurotrophic factor family.

Translocations resulting in fusion genes with several partners have been reported in lung cancer, including multiple variants of KIF5B-RET, CCDC6-

RET, NCOA4-RET and TRIM33-RET. All fusion proteins contain coiled-coil domains involved in protein dimerization. Of the different fusion proteins, KIF5B-RET is the most common (90%). RET fusion occur in 0.6-2% of NSCLCs and in 1.2-2% of AdCs, more frequently in never smokers than ever smokers. Patients with a RET fusion gene-harboring tumor are usually younger than patients with an EGFR mutation and have an equal gender distribution. RET fusion proteins have been detected in AdC and in adenosquamous carcinoma. Histological patterns that have been reported in carcinoma with RET abnormalities include those with mucinous histology or with signet-ring cells with a cribriform or solid growth pattern. TTF-1 ICH may be positive. RET gene translocations can be visualized by FISH break-apart analysis. Currently, AdCs with a RET fusion are treated in a trial context.

ROS1

ROS1 codes for a receptor tyrosine kinase of the insulin receptor family and chromosomal translocations are responsible for the occurrence of fusion genes. The prevalence of ROS1 fusions in NSCLC varies from 0.9 to 3.7%. Patients with ROS1-aberrant tumors tend to be younger than those with ROS1 wild-type tumors (median age 49.8). They are never smokers and have a tumor with AdC histology. There is no gender difference. ROS1 aberrations have also been documented in large-cell carcinoma and occasionally in squamous cell carcinoma.

KRAS

Although KRAS mutations are the oldest driven mutations known in lung cancer, they are currently not used for treatment prediction.

PIK3CA

Mutations in PIK3CA occur more often in SqCC (2-4%) than in AdC(<2%) and are associated with a poor prognosis. In NSCLC, amplification of PIK3CA is less common than mutation.

FGFR1

FGFR1 may become the first predictive marker in SqCC. FGFR1 is amplified in 10-22% of SqCC. Amplification of FGFR1 is mostly determined by FISH. Recently, an RT-PCR for amplification has been described bridging exons 14-15 and 18-19. Overexpression/amplification is associated in in-vitro studies with sensitivity to FGFR1 inhibitor.

MET

Overexpression of MET is a poor prognostic indicator in NSCLC. MET amplification has emerged as one of the critical events for acquired resistance in EGFR-mutated lung AdCs refractory to EGFR-TKIs.

PTEN

Inactivation of PTEN is due to hypermethylation, mutations or allele loss, and it leads to activation of AKT/protein kinase B independent of ligand binding and is more common in SCC than AdC (10% vs. 2%). Reduced PTEN protein expression was reported in 74% of NSCLC. Recent speculation suggests that especially in squamous cell carcinomas, reduced expression of PTEN and increased expression of AKT may characterize a subgroup of patients amenable to targeted therapy.

NUT

NUT midline carcinoma is a recently described variant of SqCC with a specific translocation. The morphology is characterized by sheets of relatively small monotonous tumor cells with occasionally abrupt transitions to well-differentiated squamous cell carcinoma areas. This tumor has also been reported in young people and has an aggressive behavior with a very poor prognosis.

An interesting morphology observation is that neoplastic cells in NUT midline carcinoma and many other carcinomas with a driver rearrangement have a slightly enlarged nucleus with a monotonous nuclear appearance (limited nuclear pleomorphysm), such as a prostate cancer, some salivary gland-type tumors (MASC, mucoepidermoid carcinoma), and ALK-positive lung cancer. In contrast, other NSCLC and many other cancer types are characterized by prominent nuclear enlargement and pleomorphism.

Tissue Management

The extended diagnostic requirements from increasingly limited material provided by minimally invasive biopsy techniques pose major challenges for pathology. Especially in lung cancer, large tumor samples are difficult to obtain. Therefore, tissue management is essential: tissue sample size should be maximized whenever feasible. In addition, tissue handling, processing, and sectioning should be standardized to minimize waste and optimize use of tissue for staining procedures and PCR-based molecular tests (distribute samples over >1 block, make a careful initial cut, spare a section for reflex analysis, focus the diagnostic analysis). Tissue management involves several aspects, leading to targeted use of the tumor sample.

In conclusion, driver biomarkers in lung cancer (point mutations, deletions, and rearrangements) provide new avenues for therapy for these patients. Biomolecular signatures may introduce a new perspective in the assessment of patients [7]. It has been demonstrated that in lung cancer patients, specific oncogenic pathways can be expressed to a different extent according to their age cohort. As a result, the activation of these pathways can be related to early metastatic dissemination.

Approximately 60% of adenocarcinomas and 20% of squamous cell carcinomas have an identified gene signature, most of which can be targeted by specific drugs. The challenge of the future is to have a targeted treatment for each gene of the known signature.

Acknowledgments

Authors thank Ms Anna Vallerugo, MA, for the English editing.

References

[1] Firat S, Byhardt RW, Gore E. Comorbidity and Karnofksy performance score are independent prognostic factors in stage III non-small-cell lung cancer: an institutional analysis of patients treated on four RTOG studies. Radiation Therapy Oncology Group. *Int. J. Radiat. Oncol. Biol. Phys.* Oct 1;54(2):357-64.2002.

[2] Martins SJ et al. Clinical Factors and Prognosis in Non-Small Cell Lung Cancer. *American Journal of Clinical Oncology*. 22(5):453, October 1999.

[3] M.B. Hazuka, W.D. Burleson, D.N. Stround, C.E. Leonard, K.O. Lillehei, J.J. Kinzie. Multiple brain metastases are associated with poor survival in patients treated with surgery and radiotherapy *J. Clin. Oncol.*, 11 pp. 369–373, 1993.

[4] Shimada Y, Saji H, Yoshida K, Kakihana M, Honda H, Nomura M, Usuda J, Kajiwara

[5] N, Ohira T, Ikeda N., Prognostic factors and the significance of treatment after recurrence in completely resected stage I non-small cell lung cancer *Chest.* Jun;143(6):1626-34. 2013.

[6] Cadranel J et al. Impact of systematic EGFR and KRAS mutation evaluation on progression-free survival and overall survival in patients with advanced non-small-cell lung cancer treated by erlotinib in a French prospective cohort. (ERMETIC project--part 2. *J. Thorac. Oncol.* Oct;7(10):1490-502, 2012.

[7] Detterbeck F, Stage classification and prediction of prognosis: difference between accountants and speculators. *J. Thorac. Oncol.* Jul;8(7):820-2, 2013.

[8] Mostertz W, Stevenson M, Acharya C, Chan I, Walters K, Lamlertthon W, Barry W, Crawford J, Nevins J, Potti A. Age and sex-specific genomic profiles in non small cell lung cancer. *JAMA*; 303:535-43, 2010.

In: Prognostic and Predictive Response ... ISBN: 978-1-63463-545-5
Editors: V. Canzonieri and M. Berretta

Chapter 6

Prostate Cancer: Prognostic and Predictive Factors

L. Fratino[1,•], *M. C. Aquilano*[2] *and V. Canzonieri*[2]
[1]Department of Medical Oncology - CRO – Centro di Riferimento Oncologico, IRCCS, Istituto Nazionale Tumori, Aviano, Italy
[2]Department of Pathology - CRO – Centro di Riferimento Oncologico, IRCCS, Istituto Nazionale Tumori, Aviano, Italy

Abstract

Prostate cancer (PC) is the most common cancer in men, in Europe and the United States, and the third leading cause of death from cancer in European men.

Clinical factors have been used to stratify prostate cancer patients and to provide guidance on the risk of cancer progression and on treatment needs. PSA screening has led to a loss in the discriminatory power of these clinical and pathologic features; nonetheless, further research is needed to identify molecular drivers of PC which if integrated with clinical factors could improve prognostication. The research for molecular prognostic factors is particularly challenging in prostate cancer given the enormous intratumoral genomic and biological heterogeneity in most early stage PC.

• Phone: +39 434 659048, Fax: +39 0434 659370, E-mail: lfratino@cro.it.

The high incidence of PC in Western countries pleads for the investigation of means to distinguish indolent from potentially lethal prostate cancers and an early identification of patients for whom treatment is indicated.

Introduction

Prostate cancer (PC) is the most common cancer in men in Europe and the United States, and the third leading cause of death from cancer in European men [1].

The high incidence of prostate cancer in Western countries underscores the urgency to develop means to distinguish indolent form potentially lethal PCa nd a timely identification of patients for whom treatment is indicated. Traditionally, clinical factors have been used to risk stratify PC patients and to provide guidance around the risk of cancer progression and need for treatment. However, the advent of PSA screening has led to a loss in the discriminatory power of these clinical and pathologic features [2]. Thus, research has turned to the identification of molecular drivers of PC, in tumors and circulation, which could be integrated with clinical factors to improve prognostication. The research for molecular prognostic factors is particularly challenging in prostate cancer given the enormous intratumoral genomic and biological heterogeneity in most early stagePC. While clinical validation of markers remains limited, several recent additions to the field show exciting futures [3].

Adenocarcinoma of the prostate is extremely h eterogeneous, ranging from an indolent chronic illness to an aggressive rapidly fatal systemic malignancy. Prognostic variables are grouped in patient-related, tumor-related and treatment-related factors [4].

The conventional clinical and pathological prognostic factors may contribute to selecting and building decision making (because the patients with high risk of early metastasis or death, would be placed in the group of more intensive treatment and follow-up) [5].

As a range of management options are available, additional prognostic factors can be considered when determining the treatment approach for an individual patient, tumors – related and treatment-related (for example the influence of each of these factors varies depending on treatment factors such as the radiation modality or the use of concomitant androgen ablation) [4].

Genetic lesions responsible for hereditary and sporadic prostate cancer show that the origin is the increasing susceptibility to oxidative damage. One of dominant oncogene mutations for PC is the transcriptional activation of truncated ETS transcriptions factor: ERG, ETV1.The androgen receptor (AR) is active throughout the course of PC and acts as dominant mutated oncogene (as the target of gene amplification, over expression, activation of mutations). It progresses by affecting transcription factors, PI3 kinase pathway and other growth stimulatory pathways [6].

Clinical Prognostic Factors

Clinical prognostic factors are assessed by physical examination, blood tests, radiological evaluation, and include the following parameters: age of patient, volume of PC-, extracapsular extension, and seminal vesicle invasion.

Age of Patient

Age of the patients is controversial depending on the study. Age greater than 65 years was a significant predictor of distant metastases at 5 years and distant failure after radical radiation therapy than a younger age [5]. Obek et al. [7] also suggested that young age per se might be an independent favourable prognostic factor for disease recurrence after surgical radical prostatectomy. Also Freedland et al., [8] found that young men had more favorable outcomes after surgical radical prostatectomy (RP) than older men, which made younger men suitable subjects for screening.

Volume

Although tumor volume is an important factor in predicting prognosis in carcinoma of the prostate, direct and accurate estimation of tumor volume is not clinically feasible. Twelve cubic centimeters was the critical volume. Higher volumes were usually associated to extensive capsular penetration, positive surgical margins, and/or positive nodes. [5].

In two important papers, the prognostic relevance of the tumor volume is stressed as predictor of progression in early PC [9, 10].

In fine needle biopsy (FNB), objective measurement of tumor routinely reported by pathologist will not be likely an accurate indicator of the true tumor volume; moreover, a consensus regarding the best method of measuring tumor length is lacking in presence of multiple foci in a single core separated by benign intervening prostatic stroma. The discontinuous foci are often the same cancer going in and out of the plane of section. The sum of measurement of each focus is the cancer length on the core. It is recommended that, at minimum the number of positive cores be recorded [11].

Prognostic Serum Markers

The increasing importance of biomarkers in screening for PC to reduce invasive follow-up procedures is proportionally reflected in the rapidly increasing number of research publications in this field, because of the distinctive relationship between the genomic changes in the cancer cells and the disease progression [12].

Circulating Tumor Cells

The development of metastases has been considered a late event in the malignant progression but evolving evidence suggests that dissemination of primary cancer cells to distant sites might occur early in tumorigenesis [13].

The bone represents the most common location of metastatic disease in PC; therefore, early works on circulating tumor cells focused on tumor cells in the bone marrow. There are significant correlations between the presence of disseminated tumor cells and clinical-pathologic parameters such as high Gleason score or metastatic disease [14, 15, 16].

The presence of these cells in the bone marrow at the time of diagnosis is also an independent negative prognostic parameter in patients with localized PC [17].

Bone marrow aspiration is invasive for the patients, therefore, additional efforts have recently focused on detection of circulating tumor cells in peripheral blood. Using polymerase chain reaction, circulating tumor cells can be detected in the blood at the time of diagnosis as well as over the course of therapy. The presence of PSA mRNA is significantly correlated to disease progression and overall survival, and their increased number has been associated with higher Gleason score and stage [18].

Immunologic approaches to detect circulating tumor cells have subsequently been commercially developed, so that a system is now available to isolate single circulating tumor cells by immunomagnetic enrichment followed by fluorimetric count. The system shows that circulating tumor cells are detectable in approximately 60% of patients with androgen-independent PC [19].

Due to their potential prognostic value, the ability to better characterize circulating tumor cells plays a significance role in order to provide more informations on cancer biology and consequential data on decision making.

Clinical Risk Group and Nomograms

Combination of clinical and pathological factors represents a more powerful tool to aid in PC prognostication. Predictive power of the clinical and pathological features, when combined together, has consistently been shown to be greater than any single factor. To this regard, several published studies have developed tools, including simple risk categories, risk calculators as well as clinical nomograms [20]. The predictive power of these clinical tools to stratify PC patients according to risk factors, have been evaluated primarily in cohorts of patients following curative therapy, either radiation or prostatectomy.

Risk categories provide clinicians and patients a qualitative assessment of the likelihood of PC progression after initial therapy. One example of risk categorization is the D'Amico Risk Classification [2] that divides men into low risk, intermediate risk, and high-risk categories of progression after radical prostatectomy, based on clinical stage, biopsy Gleason grade, and preoperative levels of PSA10. The risk grouping of an individual patient by the D'Amico classification system is determined by his most clinically advanced clinical feature, rather than a summary consideration of all three features. This risk classification system has been demonstrated in independent patient populations to provide accurate prediction of recurrence after radical prostatectomy [21].

Nomograms are chart-based tools using a scoring system of clinical characteristics to estimate individualized risk of recurrence and progression. The Kattan nomogram12 is one of the most widely used for the prediction of biochemical recurrence after radical prostatectomy. It uses information on clinical stage, Gleason grade on biopsy and pretreatment PSA levels to provide predicted probability of biochemical recurrence 5 years after radical prostatectomy. It was developed in a patient cohort with primarily clinically localized, low-risk disease.

A recent study further tested the accuracy of the Kattan nomogram12 across high and low risk strata defined by the D'Amico risk classification [22]. In that study, the authors were able to confirm the nomograms predictive ability to estimate risk of recurrence for patients with high and low-risk PC. PSA recurrence is a good, but not perfect, predictor of development of distant metastases or cancer-specific mortality.

Pathological Prognostic and Predictive Tissue Factors

Actually, Gleason score, serum PSA level, and digital rectal exam (DRE) findings are the strongest prognostic markers of progression in PC. The potential new biomarkers are used particularly on prostate biopsy specimens, using protocols that are highly standardized for the processing and scoring of the biomarkers [23].

Grading

When a biopsy proven high-grade tumour is organ confined, a relatively unfavourable short-term outcome is expected even if biologic behavior is not fully predictable on the basis of either preoperative clinicopathologic data or postoperative pathologic information obtained from the radical prostatectomy specimen [24]. ISUP Consensus Conference modified the Gleason score [25], leading to a decrease in diagnosing score 6 tumors while score 7 tumors increased [26].

Some examples of Gleason score 3+4 are showed in Figure 1, whereas a focus of a very well differentiated adenocarcinoma, Gleason score 2+2, is illustrated in Figure 2. In some cases, a tertiary pattern has been refined to include the third tumor component only when the grade is of higher Gleason pattern than the primary or secondary one [27], and furthermore if < 5% of the whole tumor. In those instances where the tertiary component was >5%, it was treated as the secondary pattern [28]. However, higher tertiary pattern has prognostic significance for PC [29].

Extracapsular Extension

A study on 196 tumours by Epstein et al., [9] demonstrated that tumors with more extensive capsular penetration had a higher risk of progression than those showing focal capsular involvement.

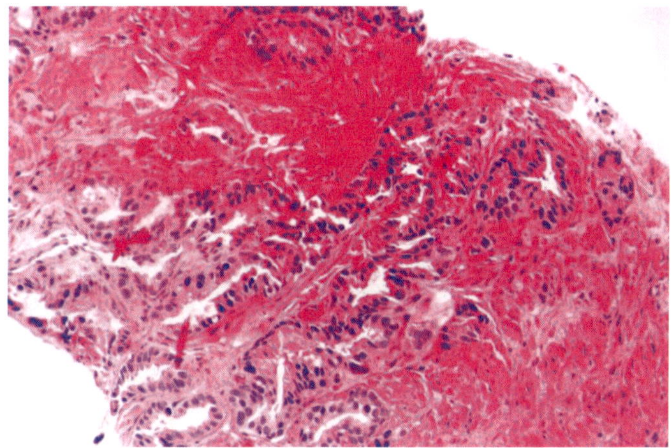

Figure 1. A focus of Gleason score 3+4 adenocarcinoma showing partial fusion of neoplastic glands.

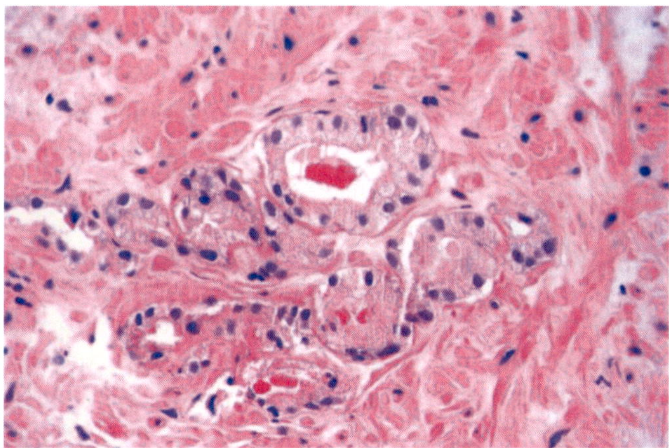

Figure 2. Few neoplastic tubules consistent with Gleason score 3+3 adenocarcinoma.

One-hundred thirty patients with more than 10- year follow-up after radical prostatectomy were histologically restaged by Theiss et al., [30].

They found that in contrast with capsular invasion as such, capsular penetration is an indicator of poor prognosis. Capsular penetration was associated to higher progression rate and reduced survival. They recommended that tumours with capsular invasion should be distinguished from those with capsular penetration. Ohori et al., [31] found that the probability of progression-free survival at 7 years was 65% for patients with extracapsular extension, positive margins, and a Gleason score of 6 or less, and 40% for patients with extracapsular extension, positive surgical margins, and a Gleason score of 7 or more.

Wheeler et al., [32] used multivariate analysis to assess the relationship between the level and extent of prostatic cancer capsular invasion, the clinical and pathological features, and prognosis of early stage PC. They found that the level of capsular invasion was an independent prognostic factor and demonstrated a strong association between the level of invasion of cancer into or through the prostatic capsule and the volume, grade, pathological stage, and the rate of recurrence after radical prostatectomy. Moreover, they concluded that sub-classification of patients according to the levels of prostatic capsular invasion provides valuable prognostic information.

Surgical Margins

Surgical margins involvement is correlated with progression, because presence of cancer within 0.1 mm of the margins confers an increased risk of (biochemical recurrence (BCR)). In these cases, adjuvant therapy should be proposed [33].

Area of Origin of the Cancer

Usually PC arises by the peripheral or transition area of the prostate gland. The cancer originating in the central area is a more aggressive form with a distinct route of spread from the gland that escapes via the ejaculatory ducts and the seminal vesicles. This cancer has a greater risk of extracapsular extension, seminal vesicles invasion, and positive surgical margins [34].

The association between the transition area tumor origin and the risk of biochemical recurrence does not add important predictive value to the standard prognostic factors [35].

Biological Prognostic Factors

Molecular pathogenesis of the PC is poorly understood. Over the past 10 years, chromosomal aberrations in PCa have been studied with several techniques (loss of heterozygosity (LOH), fluorescence in situ hybridization (FISH), comparative genomic hybridization (CGH), suppression substractive hybridization (SSH) and cDNA array hybridization). FISH has been used to identify the target genes for some of these chromosomal alterations [36]. These chromosomal alterations are most likely to harbor the critical genes for the progression of PC [37].

In general, biomolecular markers may provide useful information to better define factors that could be primarily related to aggressive and invasive neoplastic potential to spread outside the prostate [38].

E-Cadherin

E-Cadherin expression has been proposed for predicting prognosis in prostate adenocarcinoma because a study, on E-cadherin levels by immunohistochemistry in nonmalignant and malignant specimens of human prostatic tissue, revealed that patients showing low immunohistochemical expression of E-cadherin have, on average, shorter survival than patients with high immunohistochemical expression [39]. De Marzo et al. [40] correlated the down-regulation of E-cadherin and pathologic stage at radical prostatectomy.

By univariate analysis, they found that reduced levels of E-cadherin correlated with advanced Gleason score ($p = 0.003$) and advanced pathologic stage ($p = 0.008$). In multivariate analysis, E-cadherin, preoperative PSA, and Gleason score all contributed independently to the prediction of high stage disease ($p < 0.001$).

Thus, E-cadherin is considered as a potential biomarker of disease progression in patients with clinically organ-confined PC who undergo radical prostatectomy.

Moderate or strong expression of a transcriptional repressor EZH2 (enhancer of zestor homolog2) coupled with the most moderate expression of E-cadherin was the biomarker combination most strongly associated to recurrence of PC- [41].

Alpha-Catenin

Aaltomaa et al. [42] studied the expression of alpha-catenin in locally advanced PC; they found that alpha-catenin had a prognostic significance in early phases of cancer progression. Low alpha-catenin expression was related to worse prognosis than high alpha-catenin expression.

Insulin-Like Growth Factor (IGF)

The insulin-like growth factor (IGF) system is composed by two ligands (IGF-I and IGF-II), two receptors (IGFR-I and IGFR-II), and six binding proteins (IGFBP 1 to 6). Mita et al. [43] found that IGF-II and IGFBP2 play a role in PC progression, and their increased expression is a prognostic indicator in hormone- treated PC patients.

The results of the study by Figueroa and co-workers [44] indicated that the higher expression of IGFBPs in human PC correlates with the Gleason score, and the expression of certain IGFBPs may be used as markers of aggressive clinical behavior. After studying changes in IGFBP2 and IGFBP3 levels in serial postoperative serum samples from PC in patients with and without relapse, Yu et al. [45] suggested that IGFBP2 may play a role in the progression of PC but that serum levels of IGF-I and IGFBP3 have no predictive value in the progression of PC.

Androgen Receptors (AR)

The androgen receptor (AR) is a nuclear transcription factor that binds male sex steroids and mediates the biological effects of these hormones in the target cells by activating transcription of androgen-dependent genes. The AR gene is localized on chromosome X and it contains a series of CAG trinucleotide repeats. The length of CAG repeats varies among individuals and this polymorphism is believed to be related to the transcriptional activity of AR. Fewer CAG repeats are associated with increased risk of developing tumor as well as more aggressive forms of PC and breast cancer in women [46].

Segawa et al., [47] demonstrated that AR expression was significantly lower in adenocarcinoma than is non-tumor prostate tissues. They also found a significant correlation between progression free survival and AR expression or proliferative activity. High AR expression predicts high proliferative activity and short progression free survival. The greater AR heterogeneity in poor responders may reflect a greater genetic instability in tumors that have progressed toward androgen independence i.e., many of the growth factors may exhibit their effects via crosstalk with AR [48]. Magi-Galluzzi et al. [49] suggested that the heterogeneity in the expression of the androgen receptors increases with progression of invasive PCa and might in part account for variable response to endocrine therapy.

Microvessel Density (MVD)

The microvessel density count in the tumor area increases significantly with increasing Gleason score and nuclear grade [5]. The microvessel density count is a parameter under discussion among different study groups [50, 51].

p53

Thomas et al. [52] and Shurbaji et al. [53] evaluated the immunohistochemical detection of p53 protein in PC. That mutations of p53 gene, which have long half-life, are involved in carcinogenesis of PC, and that p53 reactivity marks an aggressive subset of PC. Moul et al. [54] propose to evaluate the clinical use of p53, Ki-67, and bcl2 immunohistochemical protein expression in the primary tumor as combined predictors of disease progression.

The study concluded that p53, Ki-67, and bcl2 are potential biomarkers able to predict recurrence in patients with clinically localized PC after radical prostatectomy. Grignon et al. [55] studied 471 patients assessing the statistically significant associations between the presence of abnormal p53 protein expression and increased incidence of distant metastases, decreased progression-free survival, and decreased overall survival. Among patients receiving both radiation and hormone therapies, those with tumors exhibiting abnormal p53 protein expression experienced a reduced time to the development of distant metastases.

Theodorescu et al. [56] investigated whether the levels of immunoreactivity for p53, Rb, and bcl2 are better predictors of disease specific survival than conventional pathological parameters of the primary tumour, such as Gleason's score, capsular penetration, seminal vesicle invasion, and percent of tumor in the specimen. They found that high level staining of p53 and Rb are better independent factors predicting disease specific survival than low level staining. They concluded that p53 and Rb immunohistochemical staining scores were superior to conventional pathological prognostic factors of the primary tumor as predictors of disease specific survival. Bcl-2 and p53 have been extensively examined as prognostic markers in prostate tissue, predicting the response of localized PC to radiotherapy [57].

Recently different types of p53 gene alterations have been studied [58], revealing 2 genetic subgroups with remarkable differences in their clinical course. Tumors with TP53 homozygous inactivation through deletion of one allele and disrupting translocation involving the second allele or strong p53 positivity has worst outcome, independent from clinical and pathological parameters [59].

p27

p27 is an inhibitor of the cell cycle with potential tumor suppressor function; it belongs to the Cip/Kip family of cyclin-dependent kinase inhibitory proteins down regulating cell proliferation.

Yang et al., [59] examined 86 patients with clinical stage T1-2 PCa who were treated with radical prostatectomy; they found that absence or low levels of p27 protein expression were an adverse prognostic factor in patients with clinically confined organ disease. This marker appears to be especially useful in patients with pathological stage T2-T3b disease.

p21

p21/WAF1 protein is a cyclin-dependent kinase inhibitor able to arrest the cell cycle at the G1 phase by inhibiting DNA replication.

Baretton et al. [60] demonstrated that p21/WAF1 over expression before and after androgen deprivation therapy (ADT) characterized a subgroup of advanced PCa with paradoxically high proliferation rate. Over expressing cancers had significantly worse clinical outcome than cancers with low expression level.

KPNA2

KPNA2 is associated to advanced pathological tumor stage (pT3b/pT4), high Gleason grade, and early biochemical recurrence [61].

Cell Proliferation Ki-67

Ki-67 is one of several cell-cycle-regulating proteins, which can be easily demonstrated by immunohistochemistry [62]. It is a DNA-binding protein, expressed in all phases of cell cycle but undetectable in resting cells [63]. Ki-67 index (fraction of Ki-67 positive nuclei in immunohistochemistry) is higher for carcinomas than for hyperplastic glands. Within the group of carcinomas, Ki-67 indices in patients with metastatic disease were significantly higher than in those without metastasis.

However, the results suggested that high Ki-67 index could define a group of patients with poor prognosis [64]. In another study on a group of men treated with radiotherapy and androgen deprivation for PCa , Ki-67 expression levels in conjunction with MDM2 were found to be correlated to distant metastases and survivability [65].

Urotensin II Receptor (UTR)

UTR changes occur in human prostate tumorigenesis. UTR, expressed at low intensity in hyperplastic tissue and at high intensity in well-differentiated carcinoma (Gleason 2-3) and in LNCaP androgen-dependent PC cells is considered a prognostic marker in human prostate adenocarcinoma. Korean Authors have compared a predictive nomogram for biochemical recurrence (BCR) in clinically localized PCa with Kattan nomogram.[66].

Prognostic Molecular Biology Markers

Early linkage analysis and multiple genetic variants associated to PC have now been found from genome-wide association studies (GWAS). However, their clinical utility is unknown.

Actually, the predictive biomarker candidates involving ETS gene rearrangements, PTEN inactivation, and androgen receptor are implied in clinical trials for molecular target therapy [68].

Early Prostatic Lesions

Low-grade cancer diagnosed late in life may have no impact on the quality or length of life.

There is increasing need to define molecular markers useful in men with PC- at an early stage to identify patients who would benefit from early therapeutic interventions [69].

Clinical Follow-up and Advanced Stages Management

There is no consensus regarding optimal management of localized disease. Options include watchful waiting, active surveillance, open, laparoscopic or robotic-assisted radical prostatectomy, external beam RT, and brachytherapy [70].

In men with low-risk disease, no benefit for active treatment has been demonstrated in overall survival (OS). Options for patients with intermediate-risk PCa include radical prostatectomy, external beam RT plus androgen deprivation therapy (ADT) or high-dose rate Brachytherapy [71].

In men with high-risk or locally advanced PCa, external beam RT plus hormone treatment for at least 2 years should be offered. Radical prostatectomy plus extended lymph-adenectomy can be considered in highly selected cases [I, B].Survival of PC cells depend on the activation of androgen receptors, which are over-expressed in this tumor. Furthermore, nearly 90% of PC patients responding to first-line androgen deprivation therapy (ADT) undergo rapid progression. This condition is defined as castration-resistant prostate cancer (CRPC).

In the past decade there has been a significant transformation in the cure of patients with advanced PC. New knowledge of the progression disease's mechanisms of castration resistance have generated great changes in treatment strategies particularly for patients with metastatic castration-resistant prostate cancer (mCRPC). As a result, 6 agents have been approved by the U.S. Food and Drug Administration (FDA) for targeting key disease related pathways based on overall survival advantage in the past 10 years.

For more than 40 years it was believed that advanced PCa was resistant to chemotherapy. However, two studies, TAX 3277 and SWOG 99168, independently demonstrated that docetaxel-based chemotherapy improves overall survival (OS) and health-related quality of life in men with mCRPC [72]. Docetaxel is a taxane that binds and stabilizes tubulin, inducing cell cycle arrest and inhibiting cell proliferation. Docetaxel-based regimens significantly improve survival in patients with CRPC, and represent the only treatment strategy approved by FDA The microtubule was further validated as a target in 2010, when a phase III trial demonstrated that cabazitaxel, a novel taxane, improved median OS compared with mitoxantrone (15.1 vs. 12.7 months; patients progressed on gonadal suppression are no longer responsive to hormone therapy [73].

Recently, the results of several studies have confirmed that activation of the androgen receptor is the key factor in the continued growth of PCa. The scenario of PCa treatment has changed with the approval of abiraterone –a drug that significantly reduces androgen production by blocking the enzyme, cytochrome P450 17 alpha-hydroxylase. Blockade of androgen production by non gonadal sources has led to clinical benefits in this setting.

These results have made a powerful suppression of AR signaling a prime therapeutic target in patients with CRPC. The first proof of principle was abiraterone, an oral irreversible inhibitor of the CYP- 17A enzyme, critical in extragonadal and testicular androgen biosynthesis pathway. *Abiraterone* (second hormone therapy) has been shown to improve survival in patients with CRPC who progressed after docetaxel-based chemotherapy.

Abiraterone in combination with prednisone is now approved in both post-docetaxel (2011) [74] and pre-docetaxel (2012) settings based on substantial improvement in overall survival and radiologic progression free survival (PFS) rates when compared to prednisone and placebo, respectively [75].

Another oral agent with high-affinity, selective AR inhibitor power is Enzalutamide (MDV300). Enzalutamide closely binds to the AR, decreases nuclear translocation, impairs AR binding to DNA and co-activators, and blocks cell proliferation. In 2012, Enzalutamide was approved by the FDA in the post-docetaxel setting based on results from a placebo-controlled phase III trial. The median OS was 18.4 months with Enzalutamide versus 13.6 months with placebo ($p < 0.001$), representing a 37% reduction in risk of death In the pre-docetaxel setting, another phase III trial (NCT01212991) has completed accrual, and recent public reporting of the results indicate a survival advantage

[76]. With regard to follow up, men on long-term androgen "deprivation" should be monitored for side-effects including osteoporosis.

References

[1] Malvezzi M., Bertuccio P., Levi F., La Vecchia C., Negri E. European cancer mortality prediction for the years 2014. *Ann. Oncol.,* 2014; Apr. 23.

[2] D'Amico A. V., Whittington R., Malkowicz S. B., et al. Biochemical outcome after radical prostatectomy, external beam radiation therapy, or interstitial radiation therapy for clinically localized prostate cancer. *JAMA,* 1998; 280: 969–974.

[3] Logothetis C. J., Gallick G. E., Maity S. N., Kim J., Aparicio A., Efstathiou E., Lin S. H. Molecular classification of prosate cancer progression: foundation for marker-driven treatment of prostate cancer. *Cancer Discov.,* 2013; 8: 849-61.

[4] Crook J., Ots A. F. Prognostic factors for newly diagnosed prostate cancer and their role in treatment selection. *Semin. Radiat. Oncol.,* 2013; 23: 165-172.

[5] Buhmeida A. Pythonen S., Laato M., et al. Prognostic factors in prostate cancer. *Diagnostic Pathology,* 2006; 1: 4-15.

[6] Shand R. L. and Gelmenn E. P. Molecular biology of prostate-cancer pathogenesis. *Curr. Opin. Urol.,* 2006; 16 : 123-131.

[7] Obek C., Lai S., Sadek S., Civantos F., Soloway M. S.: Age as a prognostic factor for disease recurrence after radical prostatectomy. *Urology,* 1999; 54: 533-538.

[8] Freedland S. J., Presti J. C., Kane C. J., Aronson W. J., Terris M. K., Dorey F., *et al.*: Do younger men have better biochemical outcomes after radical prostatectomy? *Urology,* 2004; 63: 518-522.

[9] Epstein J. I. Carmichael M., Partin A. W., Walsh P. C.: Is tumour volume an independent predictor of progression following radical prostatectomy? A multivariate analysis of 185 clinical stage B adenocarcinomas of the prostate with 5 years of followup. *J. Urol.,* 1993; 149: 1478-1481.

[10] Bostwick D. G., Graham S. D., Napalkov P., Abrahamsson P. A., di Sant'agnese P. A., Algaba F., et al.: Staging of early prostate cancer: a proposed tumour volume-based prognostic index. *Urology,* 1993; 41: 403-411.

[11] Epstein Ji.: Prognostic significance of tumor volume in radical prostatectomy and needle biopsy speciments. *J. Urol.,* 2011; 186: 790-797.

[12] Chikezie O., Madu and Yi Lu. Novel diagnostic biomarkers for prostate cancer. *Journal of Cancer,* 2010; 1: 150-177.

[13] de Bono J. S., Scher H. I., Montgomery R. B., et al. Circulating tumor cells predict survival benefit from treatment in metastatic castration-resistant prostate cancer. *Clin. Cancer Res.,* 2008; 14: 6302–6309.

[14] Pantel K., Brakenhoff R. H., Brandt B. Detection, clinical relevance and specific biological properties of disseminating tumour cells. *Nat. Rev. Cancer,* 2008; 8: 329–340.

[15] Wood D. P. Jr., Banerjee M. Presence of circulating prostate cells in the bone marrow of patients undergoing radical prostatectomy is predictive of disease-free survival. *J. Clin. Oncol.*, 1997; 15: 3451–3457.

[16] Berg A., Berner A., Lilleby W., et al. Impact of disseminated tumor cells in bone marrow at diagnosis in patients with nonmetastatic prostate cancer treated by definitive radiotherapy. *Int. J. Cancer*, 2007; 120: 1603–1609.

[17] Kollermann J., Weikert S., Schostak M., et al. Prognostic significance of disseminated tumor cells in the bone marrow of prostate cancer patients treated with neoadjuvant hormone treatment. *J. Clin. Oncol.*, 2008; 26: 4928–4933.

[18] Kantoff P. W., Halabi S., Farmer D. A., Hayes D. F., Vogelzang N. A., Small E. J. Prognostic significance of reverse transcriptase polymerase chain reaction for prostate-specific antigen in men with hormone-refractory prostate cancer. *J. Clin. Oncol.,* 2001; 12: 3025-3028.

[19] Goodman O. B. Jr., Fink L. M., Symanowski J. T., et al. Circulating tumor cells in patients with castration-resistant prostate cancer baseline values and correlation with prognostic factors. *Cancer Epidemiol. Biomarkers Prev.*, 2009; 6: 1904-1913.

[20] Waltz J. A normogram predicting 10 years life expectancy in candidates for radical prostatectomy or radiotherapy for prostate cancer. *J. Clin. Oncol.,* 2007; 24: 3576-3581.

[21] Boorjian S. A., Karnes R. J., Rangel L. J., Bergstralh E. J., Blute M. L. Mayo Clinic validation of the D'amico risk group classification for predicting survival following radical prostatectomy. *The Journal of urology*, 2008; 179: 1354–1360.

[22] Korets R., Motamedinia P., Yeshchina O., Desai M., McKiernan J. M. Accuracy of the Kattan nomogram across prostate cancer risk-groups. *BJU Int.*, 2011; 108: 56–60.

[23] Van der Kwast T. H. Prognostic prostate tissue biomarkers of potential clinical use. *Virchows Arch.*, 2014; 3: 293-300.

[24] Rioux-Leclercq N. C., Chan D. Y., Epstein J. I.: Prediction of outcome after radical prostatectomy in men with organ-confined Gleason score 8 to 10 adenocarcinoma. *Urology,* 2002, 60: 666-669.

[25] Epstein J. I., Allsbrook W. C., Amin M. B.: ISUP Grading Comitee. The 2005 International Society of Urological Pathology (ISUP) Consensus Conference on Gleason Grading of Prostatic Carcinoma. *Am. J. Sirg. Pathol.,* 2005; 29: 1228-1242.

[26] Helpap B., Egevad L. The significance of modified Gleason grading prostatic carcinoma in biopsy and radical nephrectomy specimens. *Virchows Arch.,* 2006; 4549: 622-627.

[27] Pan C. C., Potter S. R., Partin A. W., Epstein J. I. The prognostic significance of tertiary Gleason patterns of higher grade in radical prostatectomy speciments: a proposal to modify the Gleason grading system. *Am. J. Surg. Pathol.,* 2000: 24; 563-369.

[28] Trock B. J., Guo C. C., Gonzalgo M. L. et al., Tertiary Gleason pattern and biochemical recurrence after prostatectomy: proposal for a modified Gleason scoring system. *J. Urol.,* 2009; 182: 1364-1370.

[29] Delahunt B. et al. Gleason grading: past, present and future. *Histopathology,* 2012; 60: 75-86.

[30] Theiss M., Wirth M. P., Manseck A., Frohmuller H. G.: Prognostic significance of capsular invasion and capsular penetration in patients with clinically localized prostate cancer undergoing radical prostatectomy. *Prostate,* 1995; 27:13-17.

[31] Ohori M. et al. Prognostic significance of positive surgical margins in radical prostatectomy speciments. *J. Urol.,* 1995; 154: 1818-1824.

[32] Wheeler T. M., Dillioglugil O., Kattan M. W., Arakawa A., Soh S., Suyama K., *et al.*: Clinical and pathological significance of the level and extent of capsular invasion in clinical stage T1-2 prostate cancer. *Hum. Pathol.,* 1998; 29: 856-862.

[33] Izard J. P., True L. D., May P., Ellis W. J., Lange P. H., Dalkin B., Lin D. W., Schmidt R. A., Wright J. L. Prostate cancer that is within 0.1 mm of the surgical margin of a radical prostatectomy predict greater likelihood of recurrence. *Am. J. Surg. Pathol.,* 2014; 38: 333-338.

[34] Cohen R. J. et al. Central zone carcinoma of the prostate gland: a distinct tumor type with poor prognosis features. *J. Urol.,* 2008; 179: 1762-1767.

[35] Iremashvili V., Pelaez L., Jordá M., Manoharan M., Rosenberg D. L., Soloway M. S. Prostate cancers of different zonal origin: clinicopathological characteristics and biochemical outcome after radical prostatectomy. *Urology,* 2012; 80: 1063–1069.

[36] Nupponen N., Visakorpi T. Molecular cytogenetics of prostate cancer. *Microsc. Res. Tech.,* 2000; 51: 456-463.

[37] Pan Y., Lui W., Nupponen N., Larsson C., Isola J., Visakorpi T., Bergerheim U., Kytola S.: 5q11, 8p11 and 10q22 are recurrent chromosomal breakpoints in prostate cancer cell lines. *Genes Chromosomes Cancer,* 2001; 30: 187-195.

[38] Carter H. B., Partin A. W., Coffey D. S.: Prediction of metastatic potential in an animal model of prostate cancer: flow cytometric quantification of cell surface charge. *J. Urol.,* 1989; 142: 1338-1341.

[39] Umbas R., Isaacs W. B., Bringuier P. P., Schaafsma H. E., Karthaus H. F., Oosterhof G. O., et al.: Decreased E-cadherin expression is associated with poor prognosis in patients with prostate cancer. *Cancer Res.,* 1994; 54: 3929-3933.

[40] De Marzo A. M., Knudsen B., Chan-Tack K., Epstein J. I.: E-cadherin expression as a marker of tumour aggressiveness in routinely processed radical prostatectomy specimens. *Urology,* 1999; 53: 707-713.

[41] Rhodes D. R., Sanda M. G., Otte A. P., Chinnaiyan A. M., Rubin M. A.: Multiplex biomarker approach for determining risk of prostatespecific antigen-defined recurrence of prostate cancer. *J. Natl. Cancer Inst.,* 2003; 9: 661-668.

[42] Aaltomaa S., Lipponen P., Ala-Opas M., Eskelinen M., Kosma V. M.: Alpha-catenin expression has prognostic value in local and locally advanced prostate cancer. *Br. J. Cancer,* 1999; 80: 477-482.

[43] Mita K., Nakahara M., Usui T.: Expression of the insulin-like growth factor system and cancer progression in hormonetreated prostate cancer patients. *Int. J. Urol.,* 2000; 7: 321-329.

[44] Figueroa J. A., De-Raad S., Tadlock L., Speights V. O., Rinehart J. J.: Differential expression of insulin-like growth factor binding proteins in high versus low Gleason score prostate cancer. *J. Urol.,* 1998; 159: 1379-1383.

[45] Yu H., Nicar M. R., Shi R., Berkel H. J., Nam R., Trachtenberg J., *et al.*: Levels of insulin-like growth factor I (IGF-I) and IGF binding proteins 2

and 3 in serial postoperative serum samples and risk of prostate cancer recurrence. *Urology,* 2001; 57: 471-475.

[46] Yu H., Bharaj B., Vassilikos E. J., Giai M., Diamandis E. P.: Shorter CAG repeat length in the androgen receptor gene is associated with more aggressive forms of breast cancer. *Breast Cancer Res. Treat.,* 2000; 59: 153-161.

[47] Segawa N., Mori I., Utsunomiya H., Nakamura M., Nakamura Y., Shan L., *et al.*: Prognostic significance of neuroendocrine differentiation, proliferation activity and androgen receptor expression in prostate cancer. *Pathol. Int.,* 2001; 51: 452-459.

[48] Culig Z., Hobisch A., Cronauer M V., Radmayr C., Trapman J., Hittmair A., *et al.*: Androgen receptor activation in prostatic tumour cell lines by insulin-like growth factor-I, keratinocyte growth factor, and epidermal growth factor. *Cancer Res.,* 1994; 15: 5474-5478.

[49] Magi-Galluzzi C., Xu X., Hlatky L., Hahnfeldt P., Kaplan I., Hsiao P., et al.: Heterogeneity of androgen receptor content in advanced prostate cancer. *Mod. Pathol.,* 1997; 10: 839-845.

[50] Halvorsen O., Haukaas S., Hoisaeter P., Akslen L.: Independent prognostic importance of microvesel density in clinically localized prostate cancer. *Anticancer Res.,* 2000; 20: 3791-3799.

[51] Strohmeyer D., Rossing C., Strauss F., Bauerfeind A., Kaufmann O., Loening S.: Tumour angiogenesis is associated with progression after radical prostatectomy in pT2/pT3 prostate cancer. *Prostate,* 2000; 42: 26-33.

[52] Thomas D. J., Robinson M., King P., Hasan T., Charlton R., Martin J., et al.: p53 expression and clinical outcome in prostate cancer. *Br. J. Urol.,* 1993; 72: 778-781.

[53] Shurbaji M. S., Kalbfleisch J. H., Thurmond T. S.: Immunohistochemical detection of p53 protein as a prognostic indicator in prostate cancer. *Hum. Pathol.,* 1995; 26: 106-109.

[54] Moul J. W., Bettencourt M. C., Sesterhenn I. A., Mostofi F. K., McLeod D. G., Srivastava S., et al.: Protein expression of p53, bcl-2, and KI-67 (MIB-1) as prognostic biomarkers in patients with surgically treated, clinically localized prostate cancer. *Surgery,* 1996; 120: 159-166.

[55] Grignon D. J., Caplan R., Sarkar F. H., Lawton C. A., Hammond E. H., Pilepich M. V., et al.: p53 status and prognosis of locally advanced prostatic adenocarcinoma: a study based on RTOG 8610. *J. Natl. Cancer Inst.,* 1997; 89: 158-165.

[56] Theodorescu D., Broder S. R., Boyd J. C., Mills S. E., Frierson H. F.: p53, bcl-2 and retinoblastoma proteins as long-term prognostic markers in localized carcinoma of the prostate. *J. Urol.,* 1997; 158: 131-137.

[57] Scherr D. S., Vaughan E. D. Jm. Wei J. et al. BCL.2 and p53 expression in clinically localized prostate cancer predicts response to external beam radiotherapy. *J. Urol.,* 1999; 162: 12-16.

[58] Kluth M. et al. Clinical significance of different types of p53 gene alteration in surgically treated prostate cancer. *International Journal of Cancer,* 2014. Feb 13.

[59] Yang R. M., Naitoh J., Murphy M., Wang H. J., Phillipson J., deKernion J. B., et al.: Low p27 expression predicts poor disease-free survival in patients with prostate cancer. *J. Urol.,* 1998; 159: 941-945.

[60] Baretton G. B., Klenk U., Diebold J., Schmeller N., Lohrs U.: Proliferation and apoptosis associated factors in advanced prostatic carcinomas before and after androgen deprivation therapy: prognostic significance of p21/WAF1/CIP1 expression. *Br. J. Cancer,* 1999; 80: 546-555.

[61] Grupp K., Habermann M., Sirma H., Simon R., Steurer S., Hube-Magg C., Prien K., Burkhardt L., Jedrzejewska K., Salomon G., Heinzer H., Wilczak W., Kluth M., Izbicki J. R., Sauter G., Minner S., Schlomm T., Tsourlakis M. C. High nuclear KPNA2 expression is a strong and independent predictor of biochemical recurrence in prostate cancer patients treated by radical prostatectomy. *Mod. Pathol.,* 2014; 1: 96-106.

[62] Cooper L. S., Gillett C. E., Smith P., Fentiman I. S., Barnes D. M.: Cell proliferation measured by MIB1 and timing of surgery for breast cancer. *Br. J. Cancer,* 1998; 77: 1502-1507.

[63] Gerdes J., Li L., Schlueter C., Duchrow M., Wohlenberg C., Gerlach C., et al.: Immunobiochemical and molecular biologic characterization of the cell proliferation-associated nuclear antigen that is defined by monoclonal antibody Ki-67. *Am. J. Pathol.,* 1991; 138: 867-873.

[64] McLoughlin J., Foster C. S., Price P., Williams G., Abel P. D.: Evaluation of Ki-67 monoclonal antibody as prognostic indicator for prostatic carcinoma. *Br. J. Urol.,* 1993; 72: 92-97.

[65] Khor L. Y., Bea K., Paulus R. et al. MDM2 and Ki-67 predict for distant metastasis and mortality in men treated with radiotherapy and androgen deprivation for prostate cancer: RTOG 92-02. *J. Clin. Oncol.,* 2009; 27: 3177-3184.

[66] Cho Y. M., Jung S. J., Cho N., Kim M. J., Kattan M. W., Yu C., Ahn H., Ro J. Y. Impact of international variation of prostate cancer on a

predictive nomogram for biochemical recurrence in clinically localised prostate cancer. *World J. Urol.,* 2014; 2: 399-405.

[67] Goch C. L. and Eeles R. A. Germline genetic variants associated with prostate cancer and potentiale relevance to clinical practice. *Recent Result s Cancer Res.,* 2014; 202: 9-26.

[68] Roychowdhury S. and Chinnaiyan A. M. Advancing precision medicine for prostate cancer through genomics. *J. of Clinical Oncology,* 2013; 15: 1866-1873.

[69] Bhavsar T. et al. Molecular diagnosis of prostate cancer: are we up to age? *Semin. Oncol.,* 2013; 40: 259-275.

[70] Jones C. U., Hunt D., Mc Gowan D. G., et al. Radiotherapy and short-term androgen deprivation for localized prostate cancer. *N. Engl. J. Med.,* 2011; 2: 107-118.

[71] Wilt T. J., Brawer M. K., Jones K. M. et al. Radical prostatectomy versus observation for localized prostate cancer. *N. Engl. J. Med.,* 2012; 367: 203–213.

[72] Tannock I. F., de Wit R., Berry W. R., et al. Docetaxel plus prednisone or mitoxantrone plus prednisone for advanced prostate cancer. *N. Engl. J. Med.*, 2004; 15: 1502-1512.

[73] de Bono J. S., Oudard S., Ozguroglu M., et al. Prednisone plus cabazitaxel or mitoxantrone for metastatic castration-resistant prostate cancer progressing after docetaxel treatment: a randomised open-label trial. *Lancet*, 2010; 9747: 1147-1154.

[74] de Bono J. S., Logothetis C. J., Molina A., et al. Abiraterone and increased survival in metastatic prostate cancer. *N. Engl. J. Med.*, 2011; 21: 1995-2005.

[75] Ryan C. J., Smith M. R., de Bono J. S., et al. Abiraterone in metastatic prostate cancer without previous chemotherapy. *N. Engl. J. Med.*, 2013; 2: 138-148.

[76] Scher H. I., Fizazi K., Saad F., et al. Increased survival with Enzalutamide in prostate cancer after chemotherapy. *N. Engl. J. Med.*, 2012; 13: 1187-1197.

In: Prognostic and Predictive Response ... ISBN: 978-1-63463-545-5
Editors: V. Canzonieri and M. Berretta © 2015 Nova Science Publishers, Inc.

Chapter 7

Renal Cancer: Prognostic and Predictive Biomarkers

Carla Cavaliere[1], *Carmine D'Aniello*[2], *Sabrina Chiara Cecere*[1], *Marilena Di Napoli*[1], *Massimiliano Berretta*[3], *Renato De Domenico*[4], *Renato Franco*[5], *Michele Caraglia*[6], *Sandro Pignata*[1] *and Gaetano Facchini*[1]

[1]Uro-Gynaecologic Department, Medical Oncology Unit, Istituto Nazionale per lo Studio e la Cura dei Tumori "Fondazione Giovanni Pascale" - IRCCS, Naples, Italy
[2]Department of Oncology, Bolognini Hospital of Seriate, Seriate, Italy
[3]Departments of Gynecological Oncology Medical Oncology and Scientific Direction, National Cancer Institute, Aviano (PN), Italy
[4]Uro-Gynaecologic Department, Urology Unit, Istituto Nazionale per lo Studio e la Cura dei Tumori "Fondazione Giovanni Pascale" - IRCCS, Naples, Italy
[5]Pathology Department, Istituto Nazionale per lo Studio e la Cura dei Tumori 'Fondazione Giovanni Pascale' - IRCCS, Naples, Italy
[6]Department of Biochemistry, Biophysics and General Pathology, Second University of Naples, Caserta, Italy

Abstract

Prognostic scoring systems have been developed to stratify patients with mRCC into risk categories combining independent prognostic factors for survival. Here we described the main biological and clinical factors impacting on clinical prognostication and therapy of renal cancer.

Introduction

In the last few decades, the scientific research has focused on the investigation of molecular pathways involved in renal cell carcinoma (RCC) pathogenesis in order to better define its biology and improveclinical practice.

Several biomarkers emerged lately as prognostic and predictive tools for kidney cancer [1].

They will help to:

- Predict prognosis
- Identify patients who will benefit from a given therapy
- Minimize AEs by avoiding ineffective treatments
- Minimize cost burden on patients.

In the heterogeneous group of metastatic RCC (mRCC), the identification of these markers is required to stratify patients in homogeneous prognostic groups.

Subtypes of biomarkers are:

- Pharmacodynamicmarkers, to keep track of the pharmacologic effect of a drug (e.g. drug-related toxicity, modulation of phosphorylation of target protein)
- Prognostic markers of overall disease outcome, regardless of any specific intervention as Performance status (PS) - according to the Eastern Cooperative Oncology Group (ECOG).
- Predictive Markers of benefit or toxicity from a specific intervention (e.g. KRAS mutation as ineffectiveness of cetuximab).

A *prognostic* biomarker is a molecule that predicts survival despite any treatment; it is indicative of the innate tumour aggressiveness.

A *predictive* biomarker is a molecule that predicts therapeutic efficacy that usually implicates an interaction between the molecule and the therapy and affects patient's outcome [2].

Prognostic Biomarkers

Clinical Markers

Several prognostic scoring systems have been developed to stratify patients with mRCC into risk categories combining independent prognostic factors for survival.

Performance status (PS) - according to the Eastern Cooperative Oncology Group (ECOG) or Karnofsky is the marker with the greatest relevance. These systems highlight the impact of disease on patients overall health status, taking into account symptoms like cachexia (defined as weight loss, anorexia and fatigue) related to worse survival rates. Other clinical parameters evaluated in the scoring are the presence or absence of the primary tumour in place and any prior treatments carried out [3].

The first model, derived from a retrospective multivariate analysis, studied prognostic factors in patients with metastatic RCC treated with Interferon (IFN) enrolled in trials conducted in the 80s.

Prognostic factors included in this analysis were: the ECOG PS, the period between diagnosis and first systemic treatment, the number of metastatic sites, previous cytotoxic chemotherapies, and weight loss [4].

Based on these factors, the authors [5, 6] stratified patients in five groups with different survival rates.

Later on, in order to analyse the most important predictors of survival, many other integrated models have been designed.

The two most widely used score systems in clinical practice and trials are the MSKCC (Memorial Sloan Kettering Cancer Center) and the UISS (University of California at Los Angeles Integrated Staging System) [7].

Other clinical prognostic factors are

- Previous nephrectomy
- Time between diagnosis and therapy
- Previous RT
- Number of metastatic sites

Serum Markers

The MSKCC or Motzer criteria, evaluating 670 patients with RCC in advanced stage and treated with immunotherapy or chemotherapy, stratify patients according to five prognostic factors (two clinical markers and three serum markers) significantly correlated with overall survival (OS). The serum markers are high serum LDH (> 1.5 x ULN), low haemoglobin, high serum calcium (> 10 mg/dl) [8]. Using these variables, patients are stratified in three groups (good, intermediate and poor risk) with different prognosis, survival ranged from 20 months, for the group with a good prognosis, to 4 months for the poor prognosis one. Some laboratory parameters such as anaemia, increased neutrophil count and thrombocytosis are related to a worsening of the clinical outcome. The MSKCC prognostic risk profiles belong to the era of immunotherapy clinical trials. A subsequent validation of Motzer's prognostic scoring system to five parameters, was conducted by Mekhail and colleagues at the Cleveland Clinic and revealed some limitations, like exclusion of radiation treatments and number of metastatic sites. In this way, the addition of these parameters allows a redistribution of the patients, initially included in the intermediate prognosis group, to the group with a poor prognosis [9].

A prognostic model, adapted to patients with metastatic RCC treated with VEGF-targeted therapy, has recently been developed and is known as the International mRCC Database Consortium (IMRDC) or Heng's model. This model is derived from a retrospective study of 645 patients with metastatic RCC treated with sunitinib, sorafenib or bevacizumab plus interferon. Patients who received prior immunotherapy were also included in the analysis. The analysis identifies six clinical parameters to stratify patients into good, intermediate, and poor prognosis group.

Additional independent adverse prognostic factors validated in this model are absolute neutrophil count higher than ULN and platelets higher than ULN [10].

Table 1. MSKCC score system (Score systems)

KARNOFSKY PS	< 80%
Haemoglobin	< lower normal limit
Lactate Dehydrogenase (LDH)	1.5 x upper normal limit
Corrected Serum Calcium	> 10 mg/dl
Period from diagnosis to treatment	< 1 year

Table 2. Cleveland Clinic score system

PROGNOSIS	SCORE	Median Overall Survival (months)	Survival at 3 years(%)
GOOD	0	30	45%
INTERMEDIATE	1-2	14	17%
POOR	3-4-5	5	2%

KARNOFSKY PS	< 80%
Haemoglobin	< lower normal limit
Lactate Dehydrogenase (LDH)	1.5 x upper normal limit
Corrected Serum Calcium	> 10 mg/dl
Period from diagnosis to treatment	< 1 year
N° metastatic sites	> 1
Previous Radiotherapy	YES

Tissue Factors

Multiple prognostic factors have been studied to predict RCC recurrence including tumour stage, nuclear Fuhrman grade, histology, presence of a sarcomatoid component, micro-vascular invasion, presence of tumour necrosis and involvement of the collector system. The nuclear Fuhrman grade remains the only tissue factor considered an independent prognostic indicator for RCC [11, 12].

Histology: Clear-cell renal-cell carcinomas display divergent clinical behaviours. Several studies currently aim to identify specific molecular patterns involved in the genesis, aggressiveness and response to treatment of renal cancer. It is now widely accepted that kidney cancer, as other types of cancers, consists of different phenotypes that need different therapeutic approaches disease and patient tailored.

A pathological review of RCC revealed that more than half of the analysed samples showed deviations from classical clear cell features, suggesting that such tumours need a different classification [13, 14].

Using gene expression signatures, it is possible to discern, with more than 90% of accuracy, between clear cell, papillary and chromophobe RCCs as well as benign oncocytomas [15].

Such profiling could be an important tool in the clinical practice if validated for subtyping unclassifiable tumours or cases with unclear diagnosis (for example, eosinophilic tumours).

Furthermore, the increasing interest in neo-adjuvant therapy, makes necessary for pathologists to provide a diagnosis on limited amounts of tissue, for example core biopsies. In this case, expression profiling might be useful.

The main subtype of RCC is the clear cell one, followed by papillary type I and II, and by the chromophobe type. Many studies confirmed the prognostic value of histology and identified in clear cell carcinoma the most aggressive subtype. On the other hand, in most of the multivariate models the prognostic significance of histology loses importance in favour of tumour stage and grade [16].

Predictive Biomarkers

Clinical Factors

The onset of targeted therapy era has completely changed the scenario of mRCC treatment leading metastatic renal cancer to become the paradigm of molecular targeted therapies.

Most agents, some still in the approval phase, inhibit cellular signalling by targeting multiple receptor tyrosine kinases (RTKs). They are mostly oral small-molecules that inhibit the tyrosine kinase domain (TKI) of vascular endothelial growth factor receptor (VEGFR), platelet-derived growth factor receptors (PDGF-Rs) and other receptors such as KIT, RET, flt3 with a role in tumour angiogenesis and tumour cell proliferation [17].

The simultaneous inhibition of these targets leads to reduced tumour vascularisation, cancer cell death and tumour shrinkage. These drugs include sunitinib, sorafenib, pazopanib, axitinib and tivozanib. Another kind of inhibition is the one carried out by bevacizumab, a humanized monoclonal antibody that binds vascular endothelial growth factor A (VEGF-A).The mammalian target of rapamycin (mTOR) inhibitors, temsirolimus and everolimus, are also approved in this setting.In this context, the analysis of molecular markers, as predictive factors, may lead to a rational selection of patients able to benefit from a kind of therapy rather than another one.

Treatment selection is currently based on clinical parameters such as selection criteria for prognostic risk developed by the Memorial Sloan-

Kettering Cancer Center and based primarily on progression free survival (PFS) and overall survival (OS) data reported in phase III clinical trial [18].

However, these selection criteria appear limited and there is little data to guide the choice of drug to use.

The different selectivity and pharmacodynamics effects on receptors explain the side effects reported by each drugs.

Adverse events, commonly reported, are gastrointestinal, cardiologic, endocrinological and dermatological.

The occurrence of these adverse events, concerning the agent's mechanism of action, is due to the inhibition of target receptors, such as VEGFR (on-target effects) and to the interactions with other tyrosine kinase receptors (off-target interactions) [19].

Many studies reveal that the development of some drug-induced adverse events may be considered as a surrogate marker of its clinical activity and has a predictive value for treatment outcome.

The side effect, in this context, would be related to a major exposure to the drug and therefore it represents a marker for its increased efficacy. On the opposite, the absence of side effects would be related to sub-therapeutic levels of circulating drug leading to less therapeutic effects.

Specific adverse events, now under validation are hypertension, hypothyroidism, hand-foot syndrome and fatigue [20].

Hypertension (HTN) is an on-target effect of the vascular endothelial growth factor pathway inhibitors and the most common adverse event in patients with solid tumours treated with these drugs.

However, the pathological mechanism by which VEGF-pathway inhibition leads to an increase in blood pressure (BP) is not completely clarified; impaired angiogenesis seems to be the principal responsible for altered BP due to a generalised dysfunction of microcirculation.

Other pathways implicated are activation of the endothelin-1 system, suppression of the renin-angiotensin system, inhibition of endothelial nitric oxide synthase and increased vascular stiffness [21-23]. Many studies have focused on the association of sunitinib-induced HTN and its antitumor efficacy in patients with metastatic renal cell carcinoma. Across these studies, the incidence of all-grade and grade 3/4 hypertension varies widely according to the different inhibition ability of various VEGF inhibitors, between different protocols for measuring blood pressure used in different trials and on the basis of differences in the study patient populations [24-29].

A retrospective review from three multi-centric clinical trials, included a population of advanced and metastatic clear-cell RCC treated with sunitinib in first- or second line [9, 17 and 18], found out a significant association between sunitinib-induced hypertension and PFS, OS and objective response rate (ORR) improvement [30].The onset was early, with most cases reported before the end of cycle 2.

Hypertension is associated with a fourfold improvement in PFS and OS and a six fold improvement in ORR with sunitinib.

In the case of BP impairment, the use of anti-hypertensive drugs and/or sunitinib dosage reductions do not seem to affect the clinical outcome of patients who develop hypertension during treatment.

Furthermore, the use of antihypertensive medications at the baseline is associated with statistically significant greater OS; in fact, patients with normal blood vessel morphology may be particularly sensitive to VEGF blockade [30].

Nevertheless, it is important to have an optimal management of hypertension to prevent further cardiovascular or renal complications.

On the other hand, while sunitinib-induced hypertension is associated with statistically improved clinical outcome across the studies, the development of hypertension is not necessary or sufficient for a clinical benefit in all patients.

This hypothesis remains to be further tested and validated in prospective trials.

Hypothyroidism is another known side effect of treatment with VEGFR TKIs and is usually mild or moderate. It is recognised as a side effect of treatment in ~14% of patients treated with these agents in clinical trials [31, 32].

The mechanism leading to VEGFR TKIs related hypothyroidism is not fully understood.

Probably it is associated with a destructive thyroiditis resulting in follicular cell apoptosis [31] with endothelial dysfunction [33, 34], inhibition of iodine uptake [35, 36] and reduced synthesis of thyroid hormone [33].

Hypothyroidism treatment consists of thyroid hormone replacement therapy to allow normalisation of thyroid-stimulating hormone (TSH) levels and resolution of symptoms.

A study by Wolter et al. [37] was the first to underline a possible association between sunitinib outcome and thyroid dysfunction in 40 patients with advanced RCC. This study recorded a median PFS of 10.3 and 3.6 months and a median OS of 18.2 and 6.6 months respectively in patients with thyroid dysfunction and normal thyroid function.

In addition, a multivariate analysis showed that the development of subclinical hypothyroidism within the first 2 months of treatment was an independent predictor of survival.

In any case, larger prospective studies are needed to analyse the possible association between development of hypothyroidism and clinical outcome in RCC avoiding the bias represented by hormone supplementation in patients with subclinical hypothyroidism [38-39].

Inthis regard a prospective study of 111 patients with mRCC treated with sunitinib did not find any association between abnormal thyroid function and PFS [40] with no significantly difference between patients with and without thyroid dysfunction (18.9 versus 15.9 months, respectively) independently of line of therapy or risk status. In this study, patients were treated with hormone replacement therapy.

Hand–foot syndrome (HFS) of any grade was reported in up to 51% of patients treated with TKIs, and only in up to 9% of cases is of grade 3.

Its pathogenesis is related to the blockade of VEGFR and platelet-derived growth factor receptor with effects on dermal endothelial cells resulting in endothelial cell apoptosis. Another possible cause can be c-KIT inhibition. TKIs in fact, may have a direct toxic effect when secreted into the eccrine glands of the skin that are rich in c-KIT [41-43].

A retrospective analysis of prospective clinical trials, including patients treated with sunitinib, found out that HFS development was related to a better clinical outcome with longer OS, PFS and better ORR [44].

On this basis, HFS remains a significant independent predictor of PFS and OS [45].

Fatigue is a common side effect reported in patients receiving a TKIs therapy. It may be due to different factors directly related to the disease or not, like use of co-medications, anaemia or hypothyroidism.

In a review of clinical trials, fatigue of any grade was reported in 19%–54% of patients with mRCC treated with target therapy [46].

Other studies, investigating the role of fatigue as a predictive factor, showed that the development of asthenia/fatigue might be related to longer drug exposure. It is important to note that, even if prospective validation is required, patients who develop fatigue or asthenia have statistically significantly better clinical outcomes in terms of PFS and OS [45, 47].

Also after a multivariate analysis, fatigue or asthenia remain independent predictors for outcomes and could be related to hypopituitarism [48].

Pneumonitis are the most serious side effect of mTOR inhibitors and are probably due to a hypersensitivity response [49, 50].

This effect occurs in 2%-29% of patients with mRCC treated with temsirolimus. This range reflects the different diagnostic system used in each study (according to symptoms, it is diagnosed in 2-5% of patients, according to radiology it is diagnoses in 29% of patients) [51-53].

Similar findings have been reported with everolimus, the range was 6% to 13% in clinical trials [54, 55], and 54% in a radiographic review [56].

Data suggests that the incidence of pneumonitis may be higher in Asian patients than other ethnicities [57].

Pneumonitis may be a marker of therapeutic benefit in patients treated with mTOR inhibitors. In a review of clinical data among patients with pneumonitis, 86% achieved stable disease and 14% had progressive disease.

Of those without pneumonitis, 44% had stable disease and 56% had progressive disease.

Other Potential Biomarkers

Other common adverse events mTOR inhibitors treatment related are metabolic disorders such as increase in serum cholesterol, triglyceride and glucose levels [58].

The value of their change in serum as a predictor of temsirolimus and everolimus efficacy is under investigation.

Preliminary studies suggested that an increase in cholesterol levels, and not glucose or triglycerides, was associated with longer OS and PFS, while other studies did not confirm this predictive role.

At present, hypertension is one of the most promising and well-studied predictive clinical factors in RCC for treatment with VEGF inhibitors.

HFS and thyroid dysfunction have a potential value as useful biomarkers.

However, further investigation is required to determine the reliability of the association between the development of symptoms and clinical outcome and the possible bias related to its pharmacological therapeutic management.

Genetic Factors

Many potential candidate biomarkers for RCC among genetic factors have been studied in literature, but none of them has progressed beyond the discovery phase [59].

The expression of some genes and the presence or absence of single nucleotide polymorphisms (SNPs) have been associated with a differential response to targeted agents.

Many markers are currently in a validation phase for their possible correlation with clinical outcome.

These include genetic alterations and expression of different proteins.

Some studies suggest that SNPs in VEGFR3, CYP3A5*1, IL8, FGFR2, NR112 and ABCB1 may predict efficacy and tolerability.

However there are currently insufficient prospective data to support the use of any molecular biomarker in the clinical practice and we need appropriate trials for their validation in guiding personalised treatments.

The second-generation DNA sequencing technologies allow us to scan for thousands of somatic mutations that can be found in adult cancers.

Some of the mainly studied genetic markersin RCC include:

- Von Hippel-Lindau tumour suppressor mutations
- PBRM 1
- BAP 1
- VEGF single nucleotide polymorphisms and pathway markers

More than 90% of sporadic clear cell renal cell carcinomas (ccRCC) present *a loss of function* of VHL, a tumour suppressor gene located on chromosome 3p.

This mutation leads to stabilisation of hypoxia-inducible factors, a nuclear transcription factors that inactivate the transcription of many genes including those encoding for vascular endothelial growth factor (VEGF) and platelet derived growth factor (PDGF). The VHL gene is often inactivated (by mutation or promoter hyper-methylation) in renal cell carcinoma but its correlation with therapeutic outcome is unclear.In a study, Choueiri TK et al. [60], analysed patients with mRCC who received vascular endothelial growth factor targeted therapies. The study provided a stratification based on patients characteristics, VHL gene status and clinical outcome. The primary endpoint was the response rate correlated to VHL inactivation; progression-free survival and overall survival were investigated as secondary endpoint.

Patients with VHL inactivation had a response rate of 41% vs. 31% for those with wild-type VHL (p value = 0.34). Patients, with loss of function mutations (frameshift, nonsense and splice and in-frame deletions/insertions), had 52% response rate vs. 31% with wild-type VHL.

At the multivariate analysis, the presence of a loss of function mutations remained an independent prognostic factor associated with improved response, although PFS and OS were not significantly higher.

Another tumour suppressor gene recently implicated in ccRCC is the SW1/SNF chromatin remodelling complex gene polybromo1 (PBRM1-also known as BAF180), and its truncating occurs in 41% of the 227 cases tested [61].

PBRM1 mutations are the second most frequent event in ccRCC, ranging from 30-50% [62, 63].

PBRM1 participates in several cellular processes such as gene transcription, DNA repair and cell proliferation [64].

Many studies underline that the loss of PBRM1 is an essential event in ccRCC tumorigenesis and in tumour invasiveness.

Recently, a phylogenetic analysis, characterized PBRM1 mutations as an early event in the metastatic ccRCC development [65, 66]. Moreover, mutations of PBRM1 are frequently associated with the presence of small (< 4 cm) and highly invasive kidney tumours. Tumours are 6 times more likely to be classified as pT3a when a PBRM1 loss is present, and more than 10 times when mutations of the other chromatin modifiers are present.

Mutations of the BRCA1 associated protein-1 (BAP1), an ubiquitin carboxyl-terminal hydrolase, are strongly associated with adverse tumour features (e.g., higher nuclear grade, confirmed by Pena-Llopis et al.) and, more important, worse cancer-specific survival. Mutations in BAP1, with its inactivation occur in 15% of ccRCCs.

Mutations in PBRM1 and BAP1 are mutually exclusive; this suggests that their simultaneous loss may not be an advantage for the tumour. The median overall survival in the cohort with BAP1-mutant tumours was significantly shorter (4.6 years; 95% CI 2.1-7.2), than in patients with PBRM1-mutant tumours (10.6 years; 9.8-11.5), corresponding to a HR of 2.7 (95% CI 0.99-7.6, p=0.044). Patients with mutations in both BAP1 and PBRM1 had the worst overall survival. These findings allow identifying two mutation that define distinct subtypes of clear-cell renal-cell carcinoma with different clinical outcomes: 1) high-risk BAP1-mutant group 2) favourable PBRM1-mutant group [67].

BAP1-deficient tumours, unlike PBRM1 mutation are characterized by highly grade. Although these findings need to be validated by studies with longer follow up, the genetic status of BAP1 is likely to be used in risk stratification of patients who present with small ccRCC.

These data support the need for a molecular genetic classification of clear-cell renal-cell carcinoma that could guide the decisions making.

Other genetic sites evaluated, as SET domain containing protein 2 and Jumonji AT-rich interactive domain 1C, have also been studied although with a lower frequency (3%) [67].

A promising method to sub-classify ccRCC is the use of gene expression microarrays, in order to provide prognostic information, useful in the daily clinical practice. To date, studies using these tools have a small sample size with a limited number of analysed genes not yet validated.

Recent data of large genome-wide association study showed that some SNPs - Single Nucleotide Polymorphisms - might increase the risk of developing RCC [68-70].

Germ-linegenetic variations, in addition to somatic mutations within tumours, may also help to explain the differences in response and toxicity to anticancer agents.

Some studies demonstrate that the response to TKI therapy can be affected by the presence of some SNPs.

In a large study of 397 patients it was evaluated the association between pazopanib treatment and 27 polymorphisms amongst 13 genes regulating angiogenesis (VEGFA/IL-8/fibroblast growth factor 2), metabolism (cytochrome P450 (CYP) 3A4/5) and transport (ATP-binding cassette (ABC) B1). Two IL-8 polymorphisms, linked to its increased gene expression, was associated with a significantly shorter median PFS (27 weeks) versus those carrying the wild-type genotype (48 weeks) [71].

IL-8 has recently been identified as a potential driver of resistance to TKIs [72].

A second prospective study, examined response and toxicity to sunitinib in patients with ccRCC. Sixteen polymorphisms were examined in nine genes. Two VEGFR3 missense polymorphisms were associated with reduced PFS and a variant of CYP3A5*1 was associated with increased toxicity on multivariate analysis [73].

In a retrospective study of 136 patients with metastatic ccRCC treated with sunitinib, 30 SNPs in 11 genes were examined and correlated with PFS. Survival was significantly improved in relation to SNPs in CYP3A5, ligand-activated nuclear receptor NR1I3 and ABCB1, but not in VEGFR3 [74].

Other important genetic predictors of treatment response seem to be VEGF SNPs. These biomarkers have been associated with differences in OS between patients treated with sunitinib with and without VEGF 936 C/C and VEGFR2 889 G/G alleles and patients with other genotypes.

The frequency of the reported SNPs is typically low, so further validation studies are necessary. Furthermore, these results need to be confirmed in populations of different ethnicities.Many issues relating to the success of individualised cancer therapies come from the increasing knowledge that individual tumours are themselves highly heterogeneous [75]. Recent studies showed that the majority (two thirds) of mutations were not present in every region of a tumour, and a single biopsy would capture only a minority of the genetic aberrations. Furthermore, different areas of the same tumour presented a variety of favourable or unfavourable prognostic profiles [76], suggesting a possible diversity amongst biologically relevant (driver) mutations.

Such heterogeneity is common to all cancer types and potentially carries significant implications for successful biomarker validation and for delivery of personalized medicine.An additional complication is that the signature of the primary tumour may not necessarily reflect that of the metastatic sites [77].

The recent genome mapping has identified 259 genes that could be useful for predicting survival in ccRCC regardless of the traditional clinical prognostic factors, even if their validation is still far from being confirmed.

Tissue and Serum Factors

Some proteins have proven to be important for tumorigenesis and tumour progression. We can distinguish between proteins expressed by the tumour and detectable by immune-histochemical investigations of the surgical samples and proteins secreted by the tumour in the blood and detectable by analysis of the serum of patients during treatment.

Among these the most studied biomarkers are:

- VEGF - vascular endothelial growth factor
- CAIX - carbonic anhydrase IX
- CXCR4
- HIF-1α/HIF-2α - hypoxia inducible factor
- Phospho-S6
- PD-1L

Some studies identified sVEGFr-3 and VEGF-C low baseline levels as predictors of longer PFS in sunitinib treated patients.

Low as well as high baseline levels of VEGF predict longer PFS with sorafenib. Motzer et al. have recently published the results of an expression analysis of the plasma levels of VEGF and VEGFR in patients receiving sunitinib. In a population of 63 patients evaluated, the pattern of circulating levels of VEGF, VEGFR-2 and VEGFR-3 during treatment correlated significantly with ORR [78].

Other studies investigated the role of tumour carbonic anhydrase IX (CAIX) expression to predict the outcome in patients with mRCC treated with VEGF inhibitors. The endpoint was the analysis of the interaction between treatment with sorafenib or sunitinib and CAIX status and its impact on tumour shrinkage.

Tumour response to sunitinib or sorafenib according to CAIX status was heterogeneous without prognostic value in this setting of patients. It might be, instead, a predictive biomarker for response to sorafenib treatment. However, patients with a higher clear-cell component in their tumours were likely to have a major clinical benefit from VEGF-targeted therapy [79].

Almost 30% of the sunitinib-treated patients for metastatic renal carcinoma (mRCC) do not receive a clinical benefit.

Evidences demonstrated a cross talk between the VEGF and CXCR4 pathways and hypothesized that CXCR4 expression in primary renal cancer could predict sunitinib responsiveness.

D'Alterio et al. included sixty-two mRCC patients receiving sunitinib as first-line and evaluated the CXCR4 expression through immunohistochemistry (IHC) [80]. Correlations between CXCR4 expression, baseline patients and tumour characteristics were studied. It was detected a correlation between high CXCR4 expression and poor response to sunitinib in metastatic renal cancer. These findings, together with the ones shown by Guo J et al. allow us to draw these conclusions:

- High CXCR4 expression correlates with poor response to sunitinib
- Patients treated with sorafenib with low or no CXCR4 expression have higher PFS (20.0+5.9 mo.) than those with intermediate or high CXCR4 (6.0+0.8 mo.) (pv =.038)
- There is no correlation between low or no CXCR4 expression and PFS in patients treated with sunitinib [81].

Other scientific evidences showed that patients with higher levels of HIF-1α or HIF-2α were more likely to achieve complete response (CR) or partial response (PR) with sunitinib therapy.

Patients, with high Phospho-S6 levels versus those with intermediate or low S6 expression, showed a median OS of 17.3 versus 9.1 months when treated with temsirolimus [82].

RCC is a heterogeneous tumour that involves several molecular pathways in its development so it is difficult to predict individual response to treatment and clinical benefit.

The main difficulty for the definition of specific and generalized tumour characteristics concerns the intra-tumour heterogeneity and the lack of tumour specimens for translational research.

Our hope is to be able to use such biomarkers for early identification of responding patients.

Nowadays there are many current RCC Biomarker Initiatives:

- CAGEKID – Cancer Genomics of the Kidney [EU]
- – Genetic, epigenetic and transcriptomic analysis in clear-cell RCC
- TCGA – Tumour Cancer Genome Atlas [US]
- – Genomic profiling of tumour types (including clear-cell RCC and papillary RCC)
- Biomarker Pipeline – NIHR programme [UK]
- – Sample bank (600 patients at baseline, 200 longitudinal, long-term follow-up in all)
- EuroTARGET – TArgeted therapy in Renal cell cancer: GEnetic and Tumour related

Biomarkers for response and toxicity [EU]

- – Identify predictive biomarkers (response, toxicity) for targeted therapy
- PREDICT Consortium – Personalized RNA Interference to Enhance the Delivery of

Individualised Cytotoxic and Targeted therapeutics [EU]

- – Predictive biomarkers of response to sunitinib and everolimus
- SCOTRRCC – Scottish Collaboration On Translational Research into RCC
- – Sample bank

Clinical Follow-up

Nephrectomy is the usual treatment in localized disease; however, RCC recurs in 20-40% of patients after radical surgery. Currently there does not exist a consensus surveillance protocol. There are not prospective randomized trials in literature indicating precisely the correct timing of surveillance [83-89]. In clinical practice it is usually performed a risk-adapted approach with different protocols, according to the specialist´s experience, but not validated by any clinical study. Most follow-up protocols consider the risk of relapse in relation to the initial stage of the disease.

The high rate of recurrence for clinically localized disease after nephrectomy underscores the importance of post-surgical surveillance.

The improved survival, thanks to the availability of many new drugs to treat recurrent disease, makes necessary an early relapse detection.

Multiple prognostic factors have been studied to help predict RCC recurrence, including tumour stage, nuclear grade, overall performance status and molecular markers.

Tumour stage plays an important role in timing of recurrence.

A retrospective study stratified 559 patients with regard to T and performance status into three risk categories (low: T1, G1-2, ECOG 0; High: T3-4, G1-4, ECOG 0-3; intermediate: cases remaining):the following recommendations were produced [90]

- Low-risk patients: annual check-up with blood tests, chest x-Ray and abdominal ultrasonography,
- Intermediate-risk patients: Six-monthly check-up with blood tests and total body CT scan for 5 years followed by annual visit; follow-up could be extended to 10 years,
- High-risk patients: Six-monthly check-up with blood testsand total body CT scan for 5 years followed by annual visit for 10 years.

The greatest risk of recurrence for RCC occurs within the first 5 years after nephrectomy. The optimal follow-up duration is not defined, but it seems not to be cost effective after 5 years.

There are no studies in literature concerning the follow-up of patients with hereditary RCC. Hereditary tumours seem to have a low metastatic potential compared to sporadic tumours and it seems that the risk of metastasis increases with tumour size (T> 3 cm).

References

[1] Ravaud, A., Schmidinger, M. Clinical biomarkers of response in advanced renal cell carcinoma. *Ann. Oncol*. 2013 Aug. 7.

[2] Michaelson, M. D., Stadler, W.M.Predictive markers in advanced renal cell carcinoma.*Semin. Oncol*. 2013 Aug.;40(4):459-64. Review.

[3] Cindolo, L., Patard, J. J., Chiodini, P., Schips, L., Ficarra, V., Tostain, J., de La Taille, A., Altieri, V., Lobel, B., Zigeuner, R. E., Artibani, W., Guillé, F., Abbou, C. C., Salzano, L., Gallo, C. Comparison of predictive accuracy of four prognostic models for nonmetastatic renal cell carcinoma after nephrectomy: a multicenter European study.*Cancer* 104:1362-1371, 2005.

[4] Frank, I., Blute, M. L., Cheville, J. C., Lohse, C. M., Weaver, A. L., Zincke, H.An outcome prediction model for patients with clear cell renal cell carcinoma treated with radical nephrectomy based on tumor stage, size, grade and necrosis: the SSIGN score. *J. Urol*. 168:2395-2400, 2002.

[5] Elson, P. J., Witte, R. S., Trump, D. L.Prognostic features for survival in patients with recurrent or metastatic renal cell carcinoma. *Cancer Res*. 1988, 48, 7310-7313.

[6] Motzer, R. J., Mazumdar, M., Bacik, J., et al. Effect of cytokine therapy on survival for patients with advanced renal cell carcinoma. *J. Clin. Oncol*. 2000, 18, 1928-1935.

[7] Zisman, A., Pantuck, A. J., Wieder, J.,Wieder, J., H. Chao D., Dorey, F., Said, J. W., B. deKernion J.,A. Figlin R., and S. Belldegrun A.Risk group assessment and clinical outcome algorithm to predict the natural history of patients with surgically resected renal cell carcinoma. *J. Clin. Oncol*. 2002, 20, 4559-4566.

[8] Patard, J. J., Kim, H. L., Lam, J. S.,Dorey, F. J., Pantuck, A. J., Zisman, A., Ficarra, V., Han, K. R., Cindolo, L., De La Taille, A., Tostain, J., Artibani, W., Dinney, C. P., Wood, C. G., Swanson, D. A., Abbou, C. C., Lobel, B., Mulders, P. F., Chopin, D. K., Figlin, R. A., Belldegrun, A. S.Use of the University of California Los Angeles integrated staging system to predict survival in renal cell carcinoma: an international multicenter study.*J. Clin. Oncol*. 2004, 22, 3316-3322.

[9] Motzer, R. J., Hutson, T. E., Tomczak, P., Michaelson, M. D., Bukowski, R. M., Oudard, S., Negrier, S., Szczylik, C., Pili, R., Bjarnason, G. A., Garcia-del-Muro, X., Sosman, J. A., Solska, E., Wilding, G., Thompson, J. A., Kim, S. T., Chen, I., Huang, X., Figlin, R.

A.Sunitinib versus interferon-alfa (IFN-a) as first-line treatment of metastatic renal cellcarcinoma (mRCC): Updated results and analysis of prognostic factors. *J. Clin. Oncol.* 2009; 27: 3584-3590.

[10] Motzer, R. J., Hutson, T. E., Tomczak, P., Michaelson, M. D., Bukowski, R. M., Oudard, S., Negrier, S., Szczylik, C., Pili, R., Bjarnason, G. A., Garcia-del-Muro, X., Sosman, J. A., Solska, E., Wilding, G., Thompson, J. A., Kim, S. T., Chen, I., Huang, X., Figlin, R. A.Overall survival and updated results for sunitinib versus interferon alfa in first-line treatment of patients with metastatic renal cell carcinoma.*J. Clin. Oncol.* 2009 Aug. 1; 27(22):3584-90.

[11] Janzen, N. K., Kim, H. L., Figlin, R. A., Belldegrun, A. S. Surveillance after radical or partial nephrectomy for localized renal cell carcinoma and management of recurrent disease.*Urol. Clin. North Am.* 30:843-852, 2003.

[12] Sandock, D. S., Seftel, A. D., Resnick, M. I. A new protocol for the follow-up of renal cell carcinoma based on pathological.*J. Urol.* 1995 Jul.; 154(1):28-31.

[13] Valera, V. A., Merino, M. J. Misdiagnosis of clear cell renal cell carcinoma. *Nat. Rev. Urol.* 2011; 8:321-333.

[14] Reuter, V. E., Tickoo, S. K. Differential diagnosis of renal tumours with clear cell histology. *Pathology*. 2010; 42:374-383.

[15] Sanford, T., Chung, P. H., Reinish, A., Valera, V., Srinivasan, R., Linehan, W. M., Bratslavsky, G. Molecular sub-classification of renal epithelial tumors using meta-analysis of gene expression microarrays. *PLoS One*. 2011; 6:e21260.

[16] Vasudev, N. S., Selby, P. J., Banks, R. E. Renal cancer biomarkers: the promise of personalized care.*BMCMed*. 2012; 10:112.

[17] Motzer, R. J., Rini, B. I., Bukowski, R. M., Curti, B. D., George, D. J., Hudes, G. R., Redman, B. G., Margolin,K. A., Merchan, J. R., Wilding, G., Ginsberg, M. S., Bacik, J., Kim, S. T., Baum, C. M., Michaelson, M. D. Sunitinib in patients with metastatic renal cell carcinoma. *JAMA* 2006; 295: 2516-2524.

[18] Motzer, R. J., Michaelson, M. D., Redman, B. G., Hudes, G. R., Wilding, G., Figlin, R. A., Ginsberg, M. S.,Kim, S. T., Baum, C. M., DePrimo, S. E., Li, J. Z., Bello, C. L., Theuer, C. P., George, D. J., Rini, B. I.Activity of SU11248, a multitargeted inhibitor of vascular endothelial growth factor receptor and platelet derived growth factor receptor, in patients with metastatic renal cell carcinoma.*J. Clin. Oncol.* 2006; 24: 16-24.

[19] Tomita, Y., Shinohara, N., Yuasa, T. Overall survival and updated results from a phase II study of sunitinib in Japanese patients with metastatic renal cell carcinoma. *Jpn. J. Clin. Oncol.* 2010; 40: 1166-1172.

[20] Gore, M. E., Szczylik, C., Porta, C., Bracarda, S., Bjarnason, G. A., Oudard, S., Hariharan, S., Lee, S. H.,Haanen, J., Castellano, D., Vrdoljak, E., Schöffski, P., Mainwaring, P., Nieto, A., Yuan, J., Bukowski, R.Safety and efficacy of sunitinib for metastatic renal-cell carcinoma: an expanded-access trial. *Lancet Oncol.* 2009; 10: 757-763.

[21] Veronese, M. L., Mosenkis, A., Flaherty, K. T., Gallagher, M., Stevenson, J. P., Townsend, R. R.,O'Dwyer, P. J.Mechanisms of hypertension associated with BAY 43-9006. *J. Clin. Oncol.*2006; 24: 1363-1369.

[22] Lee, S., Chen, T. T., Barber, C. L., Jordan, M. C., Murdock, J., Desai, S., Ferrara, N., Nagy, A., Roos, K. P.,Iruela-Arispe, M. L.Autocrine VEGF signaling is required for vascular homeostasis. *Cell* 2007; 130: 691-703.

[23] Kappers, M. H., van Esch, J. H., Sluiter, W., Sleijfer, S., Danser, A. H., van den Meiracker, A. H. Hypertension induced by the tyrosine kinase inhibitor, sunitinib, is associated with increased circulating endothelin-1levels. *Hypertension* 2010; 56: 675-681.

[24] Bono, P., Rautiola, J., Utriainen, T., Joensuu, H.Hypertension as predictor of sunitinib treatment outcome in metastatic renal cell carcinoma. *Acta Oncol.* 2011; 50: 569-573.

[25] Szmit, S., Langiewicz, P., Zlnierek, J., Nurzyński, P., Zaborowska, M., Filipiak, K. J., Opolski, G., Szczylik, C.Hypertension as a predictive factor for survival outcomes in patients with metastatic renal cell carcinoma treated with sunitinib after progression on cytokines. *Kidney Blood Press. Res.* 2011; 35: 18-25.

[26] Escudier, B., Bellmunt, J., Negrier, Bajetta, E., Melichar, B., Bracarda, S., Ravaud, A., Golding, S., Jethwa, S., Sneller, V.Phase III trial of bevacizumab plus interferon alfa-2a in patients with metastatic renal cell carcinoma (AVOREN): final analysis of overall survival. *J. Clin. Oncol.* 2010; 28: 2144-2150.

[27] Rini, B. I., Halabi, S., Rosenberg, J. E., Stadler, W. M., Vaena, D. A., Archer, L., Atkins, J. N., Picus, J., Czaykowski, P., Dutcher, J., Small, E. J.Phase III trial of bevacizumab plus interferon alfa versus interferon alfa monotherapy in patients with metastatic renal cell carcinoma: final results of CALGB 90206. *J. Clin. Oncol.* 2010; 28: 2137-2143.

[28] Rini, B. I., Escudier, B., Tomczak, P., Kaprin, A., Szczylik, C., Hutson, T. E., Michaelson, M. D., Gorbunova, V. A., Gore, M. E., Rusakov, I. G., Negrier, S., Ou, Y. C., Castellano, D., Lim, H. Y., Uemura, H., Tarazi, J., Cella, D., Chen, C., Rosbrook, B., Kim, S., Motzer, R. J. Comparative effectiveness of axitinib versus sorafenib in advanced renal cell carcinoma (AXIS): a randomised phase 3 trial.*Lancet* 2011; 378: 1931-1939.

[29] Nosov, D. A., Esteves, B., Lipatov, O. N., Lyulko, A. A., Anischenko, A. A., Chacko, R. T., Doval, D. C., Strahs, A., Slichenmyer, W. J., Bhargava, P.Antitumor activity and safety of tivozanib (AV-951) in a phase II randomized discontinuation trial in patients with renal cell carcinoma. *J. Clin. Oncol.* 2012; 30: 1678-1685.

[30] Rini, B. I., Cohen, D. P., Lu, D. R., Chen, I., Hariharan, S., Gore, M. E., Figlin, R. A., Baum, M. S., Motzer, R. J.Hypertension as a biomarker of efficacy in patients with metastatic renal cell carcinoma treated with sunitinib.*J. Natl. Cancer Inst.* 2011 May 4; 103(9):763-73. Epub. 2011 Apr. 28.

[31] Rini, B. I., Tamaskar, I., Shaheen, P. Hypothyroidism in patients with metastatic renal cell carcinoma treated with sunitinib. *J. Natl. Cancer Inst.*2007; 99: 81-83.

[32] Wolter, P., Dumez, H., Schoffski, P. Sunitinib and hypothyroidism. *N. Engl. J. Med.* 2007; 356: 1580-1581.

[33] Wong, E., Rosen, L. S., Mulay, M., Vanvugt, A., Dinolfo, M., Tomoda, C., Sugawara, M., Hershman, J. M.Sunitinib induces hypothyroidism in advanced cancer patients and may inhibit thyroid peroxidase activity. *Thyroid* 2007; 17: 351-355.

[34] Baffert, F., Le, T., Thurston, G.,McDonald, D. M. Angiopoietin-1 decreases plasma leakage by reducing number and size of endothelial gaps in venules. *Am. J. Physiol. Heart Circ. Physiol.* 2006; 290: H107-H118.

[35] Grossmann, M., Premaratne, E., Desai, J., Davis, I. D.Thyrotoxicosis during sunitinib treatment for renal cell carcinoma. *Clin. Endocrinol.*(Oxf.) 2008; 69: 669-672.

[36] Mannavola, D., Coco, P., Vannucchi, G., Bertuelli, R., Carletto, M., Casali, P. G., Beck-Peccoz, P., Fugazzola, L.A novel tyrosine-kinase selective inhibitor, sunitinib, induces transient hypothyroidism by blocking iodine uptake. *J. Clin. Endocrinol. Metab.* 2007; 92: 3531-3534.

[37] Wolter, P., Stephan, C., Decallonne, B. Evaluation of thyroid dysfunction as a candidate surrogate marker for efficacy of sunitinib in patients (pts) with advanced renal cell cancer (RCC). *J. Clin. Oncol.* 2008; 26 (Suppl.) (Abstract 5126).

[38] Schmidinger, M., Vogl, U. M., Bojic, M., Lamm, W., Heinzl, H., Haitel, A., Clodi, M., Kramer, G., Zielinski, C. C.Hypothyroidism in patients with renal cell carcinoma: blessing or curse? *Cancer* 2011; 117: 534-544.

[39] Pinto, A., Moreno, V., Aguayo, C., et al. Hypothyroidism and macrocytosis as surrogate markers for response and survival in patients with advanced renal cell carcinoma treatment with sunitinib as first-line therapy. *ECCO16-ESMO36-ESTRO30 2011.*

[40] Sabatier, R., Eymard, J. C., Walz, J., Deville, J. L., Narbonne, H., Boher, J. M., Salem, N., Marcy, M., Brunelle, S., Viens, P., Bladou, F., Gravis, G. Could thyroid dysfunction influence outcome in sunitinib-treated metastatic renal cell carcinoma? *Ann. Oncol.* 2012; 23: 714-721.

[41] Lacouture, M. E., Reilly, L. M., Gerami, P.,Guitart, J. Hand foot skin reaction in cancer patients treated with the multikinase inhibitors sorafenib and sunitinib. *Ann. Oncol.* 2008; 19: 1955-1961.

[42] Erber, R., Thurnher, A., Katsen, A. D., Groth, G., Kerger, H., Hammes, H. P., Menger, M. D., Ullrich, A., Vajkoczy, P.Combined inhibition of VEGF and PDGF signaling enforces tumor vessel regression by interfering with pericyte-mediated endothelial cell survival mechanisms. *FASEB J.* 2004; 18: 338-340.

[43] Yang, C. H., Lin, W. C., Chuang, C. K., Chang, Y. C., Pang, S. T., Lin, Y. C., Kuo, T. T., Hsieh, J. J., Chang, J. W.Hand-foot skin reaction in patients treated with sorafenib: a clinicopathological study of cutaneous manifestations due to multitargeted kinase inhibitor therapy. *Br. J. Dermatol.* 2008; 158: 592-596.

[44] Pusanov, I., Michaelson, D., Cohen, D. Evaluation of hand-foot syndrome (HFS) as a potential biomarker of sunitinib efficacy in patients with metastatic renal cell carcinoma (mRCC) and gastrointestinal stromal tumour (GIST). *ECCO16-ESMO36-ESTRO30 2011.*

[45] Donskov, F., Michaelson, M. D., Puzanov, I. Comparative assessment of sunitinib associated adverse events as potential biomarkers of efficacy in metastatic renal cell carcinoma (mRCC). *Ann. Oncol.* 2012; 23(Suppl. 9).

[46] Larkin, J. M., Pyle, L. M., Gore, M. E. Fatigue in renal cell carcinoma: the hidden burden of current targeted therapies. *Oncologist* 2010; 15: 1135-1146.

[47] Davis, M., Figlin, R., Hutson, T. E. Asthenia and fatigue as potential biomarkers of sunitinib efficacy in metastatic renal cell carcinoma. *ECCO16-ESMO36-ESTRO30 2011* (Abstract 1139).

[48] Wolter, P., Wildiers, D., Vanderschueren, H.Hypogonadism in male patients treated with the tyrosine kinase inhibitors sunitinib or sorafenib. *J. Clin. Oncol.* 2009; 27(Suppl. 15s) (Abstract 3565).

[49] Pham, P. T., Pham, P. C., Danovitch, G. M., Ross, D. J., Gritsch, H. A., Kendrick, E. A., Singer, J., Shah, T., Wilkinson, A. H.Sirolimus-associated pulmonary toxicity.*Transplantation* 2004; 77: 1215-1220.

[50] Morelon, E., Stern, M., Israel-Biet, D., Correas, J. M., Danel, C., Mamzer-Bruneel, M. F., Peraldi, M. N., Kreis, H.Characteristics of sirolimus-associated interstitial pneumonitis in renal transplant patients. *Transplantation* 2001; 72: 787-790.

[51] Atkins, M. B., Hidalgo, M., Stadler, W. M., Logan, T. F., Dutcher, J. P., Hudes, G. R., Park, Y., Liou, S. H., Marshall, B., Boni, J. P., Dukart, G., Sherman, M. L.Randomized phase II study of multiple dose levels of CCI-779, a novel mammalian target of rapamycin kinase inhibitor, in patients with advanced refractory renal cell carcinoma. *J. Clin. Oncol.* 2004; 22:909-918.

[52] Bellmunt, J., Szczylik, C., Feingold, J., Strahs, A., Berkenblit, A.Temsirolimus safety profile and management of toxic effects in patients with advanced renal cell carcinoma and poor prognostic features. *Ann. Oncol.* 2008; 19: 1387-1392.

[53] Maroto, J. P., Hudes, G., Dutcher, J. P., Logan, T. F., White, C. S., Krygowski, M., Cincotta, M., Shapiro, M., Duran, I., Berkenblit, A.Drug-related pneumonitis in patients with advanced renal cell carcinoma treated with temsirolimus. *J. Clin. Oncol.* 2011; 29: 1750-1756.

[54] Motzer, R. J., Escudier, B., Oudard, S., Hutson, T. E., Porta, C., Bracarda, S., Grünwald, V., Thompson, J. A., Figlin, R. A., Hollaender, N., Kay, A., Ravaud, A.; RECORD1 Study Group.Phase 3 trial of everolimus for metastatic renal cell carcinoma: results and analysis of prognostic factors. *Cancer* 2010; 116: 4256-4265.

[55] Grunwald, V., Karakiewicz, P. I., Bavbek, S. E., Miller, K., Machiels, J. P., Lee, S. H., Larkin, J., Bono, P., Rha, S. Y., Castellano, D., Blank, C. U., Knox, J. J., Hawkins, R., Anak, O., Rosamilia, M., Booth, J., Pirotta,

N., Bodrogi, I.; REACT Study Group.An international expanded-access programme of everolimus: addressing safety and efficacy in patients with metastatic renal cell carcinoma who progress after initial vascular endothelial growth factor receptor-tyrosine kinase inhibitor therapy. *Eur. J. Cancer* 2012; 48: 324-332.

[56] White, D. A., Camus, P., Endo, M., Escudier, B., Calvo, E., Akaza, H., Uemura, H., Kpamegan, E., Kay, A., Robson, M., Ravaud, A., Motzer, R. J.Noninfectious pneumonitis after everolimus therapy for advanced renal cell carcinoma. *Am. J. Respir. Crit. Care Med.* 2010; 182: 396-403.

[57] Ogura, T., Morita, S., Yonemori, K., T. Nonaka, T. Urano. Can we detect any ethnic differences in toxicity in early phase clinical trials for anticancer drugs? *ECCO16-ESMO36-ESTRO30 2011* (Abstract 1304).

[58] Lee, C. K., Marschner, R., Simes, J., Voysey, M., Egleston, B., Hudes, G., de Souza, P.Increase in cholesterol predicts survival advantage in renal cell carcinoma patients treated with temsirolimus. *Clin. Cancer Res.* 2012; 18: 3188-3196.

[59] Eisengart, L. J., MacVicar, G. R., Yang, X. J. Predictors of response to targeted therapy in renal cell carcinoma. *Arch. Pathol. Lab. Med.* 2012, 136:490-495.

[60] Choueiri, T. K., Vaziri, S. A., Jaeger, E., Elson, P., Wood, L., Bhalla, I. P., Small, E. J., Weinberg, V., Sein, N., Simko, J., Golshayan, A. R., Sercia, L., Zhou, M., Waldman, F. M., Rini, B. I., Bukowski, R. M., Ganapathi, R. Von Hippel-Lindau gene status and response to vascular endothelial growth factor targeted therapy for metastatic clear cell renal cell carcinoma.*J. Urol.* 2008;180:860-866.

[61] Varela, I., Tarpey, P., Raine, K., Huang, D., Ong, C. K., Stephens, P., Davies, H., Jones, D., Lin, M. L., Teague, J., Bignell, G., Butler, A., Cho, J., Dalgliesh, G. L., Galappaththige, D., Greenman, C., Hardy, C., Jia, M., Latimer, C., Lau, K. W., Marshall, J., McLaren, S., Menzies, A., Mudie, L., Stebbings, L., Largaespada, A.,Wessels, L. F., Richard, S., Kahnoski, R. J., Anema, J., et al. Exome sequencing identifies frequent mutation of the SWI/SNF complex gene PBRM1 inrenal carcinoma.*Nature* 2011, 469:539-542.

[62] Young, A. C., Craven, R. A., Cohen, D., Taylor, C., Booth, C., Harnden, P., Cairns, D. A., Astuti, D., Gregory, W., Maher, E. R., Knowles, M. A., Joyce, A., Selby, P. J., Banks, R. E. Analysis of VHL gene alterations and their relationship to clinical parameters in sporadic conventional renal cell carcinoma. *Clin. CancerRes.* 15:7582-7592.

[63] Nickerson, M. L., Jaeger, E., Shi, Y., Durocher, J. A., Mahurkar, S., Zaridze, D., Matveev, V., Janout, V., Kollarova, H., Bencko, V., Navratilova, M., Szeszenia-Dabrowska, N., Mates, D., Mukeria, A., Holcatova, I., Schmidt, L. S., Toro, J. R., Karami, S., Hung, R., Gerard, G. F., Linehan, W. M., Merino, M., Zbar, B., Boffetta, P., Brennan, P., Rothman, N., Chow, W. H., Waldman, F. M., Moore, L. E. Improved identification of von Hippel-Lindau gene alterations in clear cell renal tumors. *Clin. Cancer Res.* 2008, 14:4726-4734.

[64] Sun, M., Shariat, S. F., Cheng, C., Ficarra, V., Murai, M., Oudard, S., Pantuck, A. J., Zigeuner, R., Karakiewicz, P. I. Prognostic factors and predictive models in renal cell carcinoma: a contemporary review. *Eur. Urol.* 2011, 60:644-661.

[65] Motzer, R. J., Hutson, T. E., Tomczak, P., Michaelson, M. D., Bukowski, R. M., Rixe, O., Oudard, S., Negrier, S., Szczylik, C., Kim, S. T., Chen, I., Bycott, P. W., Baum, C. M., Figlin, R. A. Sunitinib versus interferon alfa in metastatic renal-cell carcinoma.*N. Engl. J. Med.* 2007, 356:115-124.

[66] Sternberg, C. N., Davis, I. D., Mardiak, J., Szczylik, C., Lee, E., Wagstaff, J., Barrios, C. H., Salman, P., Gladkov, O. A., Kavina, A., Zarbá, J. J., Chen, M., McCann, L., Pandite, L., Roychowdhury, D. F., Hawkins, R. E. Pazopanib in locally advanced or metastatic renal cell carcinoma: results of a randomized phase III trial. *J. Clin. Oncol.* 2010, 28:1061-1068.

[67] Peña-Llopis, S., Vega-Rubín-de-Celis, S., Liao, A., Leng, N., Pavía-Jiménez, A., Wang, S., Yamasaki, T., Zhrebker, L., Sivanand, S., Spence, P., Kinch, L., Hambuch, T., Jain, S., Lotan, Y., Margulis, V., Sagalowsky, A. I., Summerour, P. B., Kabbani, W., Wong, S. W., Grishin, N., Laurent, M., Xie, X. J., Haudenschild, C. D., Ross, M. T., Bentley, D. R., Kapur, P., Brugarolas, J. BAP1 loss defines a new class of renal cell carcinoma. *Nat. Genet.* 2012, 44:751-759.

[68] Dalgliesh, G. L., Furge, K., Greenman, C., Chen, L., Bignell, G., Butler, A., Davies, H., Edkins, S., Hardy, C., Latimer, C., Teague, J., Andrews, J., Barthorpe, S., Beare, D., Buck, G., Campbell, P. J., Forbes, S., Jia, M., Jones, D., Knott, H., Kok, C. Y., Lau, K. W., Leroy, C., Lin, M. L., McBride, D. J., Maddison, M., Maguire, S., McLay, K., Menzies, A., Mironenko, T., et al. Systematic sequencing of renal carcinoma reveals inactivation of histone modifying genes. *Nature* 2010, 463:360-363.

[69] Purdue, M. P., Johansson, M., Zelenika, D., Toro, J. R., Scelo, G., Moore, L. E., Prokhortchouk, E., Wu, X., Kiemeney, L. A., Gaborieau,

V., Jacobs, K. B., Chow, W. H., Zaridze, D., Matveev, V., Lubinski, J., Trubicka, J., Szeszenia-Dabrowska, N., Lissowska, J., Rudnai, P., Fabianova, E., Bucur, A., Bencko, V., Foretova, L., Janout, V., Boffetta, P., Colt, J. S., Davis, F. G., Schwartz, K. L., et al. Genome-wide association study of renal cell carcinoma identifies two susceptibility loci on 2p21 and 11q13.3. *Nat. Genet*. 2011, 43:60-65.

[70] Wu, X., Scelo, G., Purdue, M.P., Rothman, N., Johansson, M., Ye, Y., Wang, Z., Zelenika, D., Moore, L. E., Wood, C. G., Prokhortchouk, E., Gaborieau, V., Jacobs, K. B., Chow, W. H., Toro, J. R., Zaridze, D., Lin, J., Lubinski, J., Trubicka, J., Szeszenia-Dabrowska, N., Lissowska, J., Rudnai, P., Fabianova, E., Mates, D., Jinga, V., Bencko, V., Slamova, A., Holcatova, I., Navratilova, M., Janout, V., et al. A genome-wide association study identifies a novel susceptibility locus for renal cell carcinoma on 12p11.23.*Hum. Mol. Genet*. 2012, 21:456-462.

[71] Xu, C. F., Bing, N. X., Ball, H. A., Rajagopalan, D., Sternberg, C. N., Hutson, T. E., de Souza, P., Xue, Z. G., McCann, L., King, K. S., Ragone, L. J., Whittaker, J. C., Spraggs, C. F., Cardon, L. R., Mooser, V. E., Pandite, L. N.: Pazopanib efficacy in renal cell carcinoma: evidence for predictive genetic markers in angiogenesisrelated and exposure-related genes.*J. Clin. Oncol*. 2011, 29:2557-2564.

[72] Huang, D., Ding, Y., Zhou, M., Rini, B. I., Petillo, D., Qian, C. N., Kahnoski, R., Futreal, P. A., Furge, K. A., Teh, B. T. Interleukin-8 mediates resistance toantiangiogenic agent sunitinib in renal cell carcinoma. *Cancer Res*. 2010, 70:1063-1071.

[73] Garcia-Donas, J., Esteban, E., Leandro-Garcia, L. J., Castellano, D. E., del Alba, A. G., Climent, M. A., Arranz, J. A., Gallardo, E., Puente, J., Bellmunt, J., Mellado, B., Martínez, E., Moreno, F., Font, A., Robledo, M., Rodríguez-Antona, C. Single nucleotide polymorphism associations with response and toxic effects in patients with advanced renal-cell carcinoma treated with first-line sunitinib: a multicentre, observational, prospective study. *Lancet Oncol*. 2011, 12:1143-1150.

[74] Van der Veldt, A. A., Eechoute, K., Gelderblom, H., Gietema, J., Guchelaar, H. J., van Erp, N. P., van den Eertwegh, A. J., Haanen, J. B., Mathijssen, R. H., Wessels, J. A. Genetic polymorphisms associated with a prolonged progression-free survival in patients with metastatic renal cell cancer treated with sunitinib. *Clin. CancerRes*. 2011, 17:620-629.

[75] Marusyk, A., Almendro, V., Polyak, K. Intra-tumour heterogeneity: a looking glass for cancer? *Nat. Rev. Cancer* 2012, 12:323-334.

[76] Brannon, A. R., Reddy, A., Seiler, M., Arreola, A., Moore, D. T., Pruthi, R. S., Wallen, E. M., Nielsen, M. E., Liu, H., Nathanson, K. L., Ljungberg, B., Zhao, H., Brooks, J. D., Ganesan, S., Bhanot, G., Rathmell, W. K. Molecular stratification of clear cell renal cell carcinoma by consensus clustering reveals distinct subtypes and survival patterns.*Genes Cancer* 2010, 1:152-163.

[77] Gerlinger, M., Rowan, A. J., Horswell, S., Larkin, J., Endesfelder, D., Gronroos, E., Martinez, P., Matthews, N., Stewart, A., Tarpey, P., Varela, I., Phillimore, B., Begum, S., McDonald, N. Q., Butler, A., Jones, D., Raine, K., Latimer, C., Santos, C. R., Nohadani, M., Eklund, A. C., Spencer-Dene, B., Clark, G., Pickering, L., Stamp, G., Gore, M., Szallasi, Z., Downward, J., Futreal, P. A., Swanton, C. Intratumor heterogeneity and branched evolution revealed by multiregion sequencing.*N. Engl. J. Med.* 2012, 366:883-892.

[78] Rini, B. I., Cohen, D. P., Lu, D. R., Chen, I., Hariharan, S., Gore, M. E., Figlin, R. A., Baum, M. S., Motzer, R. J. Hypertension as a biomarker of efficacy in patients with metastatic renal cell carcinoma treated with sunitinib.*I* 2011;103:763-773.

[79] Choueiri, T. K.,Regan, M. M., Rosenberg, J. E., Oh, W. K., Clement, J., Amato, A. M., McDermott, D., Cho, D. C., Atkins, M. B., Signoretti, S. Carbonic anhydrase IX and pathological features as predictors of outcome in patients with metastatic clear-cell renal cell carcinoma receiving vascular endothelial growth factor-targeted therapy.*Br. J. Urol. Int.* 2010;106:772-778.

[80] D' Alterio, C., Portella, L., Ottaiano, A., Rizzo, M., Carteni, G., Pignata, S., Facchini, G., Perdona, S., Di Lorenzo, G., Autorino, R., Franco, R., La Mura, A., Nappi, O., Castello, G., Scala, S.High CXCR4 expression correlates with sunitinib poor response in metastatic renal cancer.*Curr. Can. Drug Targets*. 2012; 12:693-702.

[81] Guo, J., B. Tang, X. N. Sheng, C. L. Cui.Use of CXCR4 expression to predict the efficacy of sorafenib treatment in patients with metastatic renal cell carcinoma.*J. Clin. Oncol.* 2011; 29: abstract 359.

[82] P. H. Patel, R. S. Chadalavada, N. M. Ishill, S. Patil, V. E. Reuter, R. J. Motzer, and R. S. Chaganti. Hypoxia-inducible factor (HIF) 1 and 2 levels in cell lines and human tumor predicts response to sunitinib in renal cell carcinoma (RCC) *J. Clin. Oncol.* 2008; 26: abstract 5008.

[83] Lam, J. S., Shvarts, O., Leppert, J. T., Pantuck, A. J., Figlin, R. A., Belldegrun, A. S. Postoperative surveillance protocol for patients with localized and locally advanced renal cell carcinoma based on a validated

prognostic nomogram and risk group stratification system.*J. Urol.* 174:466-472, 2005.

[84] Leibovich, B. C.,Blute, M. L., Cheville, J. C., Lohse, C. M., Frank, I., Kwon, E. D., Weaver, A. L., Parker, A. S., Zincke, H. Prediction of progression after radical nephrectomy for patients with clear cell renal cell carcinoma: a stratification tool for prospective clinical trials. *Cancer* 97:1663-1671, 2003.

[85] Kattan, M. W., Snyder, M. E., Reuter, V., Motzer, R., Goetzl, M., McKiernan, J., Russo, P.A postoperative prognostic nomogram for renal cell carcinoma. *J. Urol.* 166:63-67, 2001.

[86] Zisman, A., Pantuck, A. J., Wieder, J., Chao, D. H., Dorey, F., Said, J. W., deKernion, J. B., Figlin, R. A., Belldegrun, A. S. Risk group assessment and clinical outcome algorithm to predict the natural history of patients with surgically resected renal cell carcinoma. *J. Clin. Oncol.* 20:4559-4566, 2002.

[87] Sorbellini, M., Kattan, M. W., Snyder, M. E., Reuter, V., Motzer, R., Goetzl, M., McKiernan, J., Russo, P. A postoperative prognostic nomogram predicting recurrence for patients with conventional clear cell renal cell carcinoma. *J. Urol.* 173:48-51, 2005.

[88] Lau, W. K.,Blute, M. L., Weaver, A. L., Torres, V. E., Zincke, H. Matched comparison of radical nephrectomy vs nephron-sparing surgery in patients with unilateral renal cell carcinoma and a normal contralateral kidney.*Mayo Clin. Proc.* 75:1236-1242, 2000.

[89] Levy, D. A., Slaton, J. W., Swanson, D. A., Dinney, C. P. Stage specific guidelines for surveillance after radical nephrectomy for local renal cell carcinoma.*J. Urol.* 159:1163-1167, 1998.

[90] Lam, J. S., Shvarts, O., Leppert, J. T., Pantuck, A. J., Figlin, R. A., Belldegrun, A. S.Postoperative surveillance protocol for patients with localized and locally advanced renal cell carcinoma based on a validated prognostic nomogram and risk group stratification system. *J. Urol.* 174:466-472, 2005.

Editors Contact Information

Dr. Vincenzo Canzonieri, Division of Pathology,
CRO Aviano National Cancer Institute IRCCS
Via Franco Gallini, 2 33081 Aviano
Tel: +390434659618
E-mail: vcanzonieri@cro.it

Dr. Massimiliano Berretta,
Division of Oncology,
CRO Aviano National Cancer Institute IRCCS
Via Franco Gallini, 2 33081 Aviano
Tel: +390434659724
E-mail: mberretta@cro.it

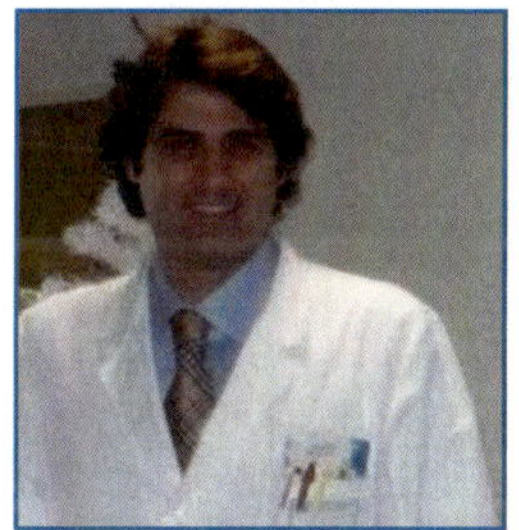

Index

D

E

F

G

H

I

J

K

L

M

Q

R

S

T

U

V

W

Y